Diagr
Mana
Rhin
Rhinosinusitis

Third Edition

James A. Hadley, MD, FACS
Associate Professor Otolaryngology
University of Rochester Medical Center

Mani S. Kavuru, MD
Director, Pulmonary Function Laboratory
Department of Pulmonary and Critical Care Medicine
Cleveland Clinic Foundation

Jack B. Anon, MD
Clinical Professor, Department of Otolaryngology
University of Pittsburgh School of Medicine

Lily C. Pien, MD
Associate Staff, Section of Allergy and Immunology
Department of Pulmonary and Critical Care Medicine
Cleveland Clinic Foundation

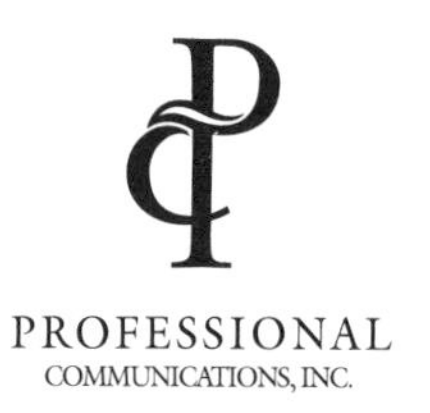

PROFESSIONAL
COMMUNICATIONS, INC.

Professional Communications, Inc.
A Medical Publishing Company

Marketing Office:
400 Center Bay Drive
West Islip, NY 11795
(t) 631/661-2852
(f) 631/661-2167

Editorial Office:
PO Box 10
Caddo, OK 74729-0010
(t) 580/367-9838
(f) 580/367-9989

For orders only, please call
1-800-337-9838
or visit our website at
www.pcibooks.com

ISBN: 1-932610-02-2

Printed in the United States of America

DISCLAIMER

The opinions expressed in this publication reflect those of the authors. However, the authors make no warranty regarding the contents of the publication. The protocols described herein are general and may not apply to a specific patient. Any product mentioned in this publication should be taken in accordance with the prescribing information provided by the manufacturer.

This text is printed on recycled paper.

DEDICATION

This reference is dedicated to my wife and children for their ever-loving support and understanding.

— JAH

We dedicate this work to the memory of our colleague, teacher, and friend, Dr. William Wagner. He will be remembered for his tireless service to his patients and the Cleveland Clinic.

— MSK
— LCP

To my wife Ellen and sons Josh and Seth for their encouragement, support, and understanding. Unleash the power, no capes, and go Trojans!

— JBA

TABLE OF CONTENTS

Introduction	1
Rhinitis: Definition, Classification, and Epidemiology	2
Rhinitis: Pathogenesis	3
Rhinitis: Diagnosis	4
Rhinitis: Nonpharmacologic Therapy	5
Rhinitis: Pharmacologic Therapy	6
Rhinitis: Immunotherapy	7
Coexistence of Rhinitis and Asthma	8
Rhinosinusitis: Definition, Classification, and Epidemiology	9
Rhinosinusitis: Anatomy and Pathophysiology	10
Rhinosinusitis: Diagnosis	11
Acute Bacterial Rhinosinusitis: Pharmacologic Therapy	12
Chronic Rhinosinusitis	13
Case Studies	14
Resources	15
References	16
Index	17

TABLES

Table 2.1 Chronic Rhinitis Syndromes 14

Table 2.2 Occupational Irritants 17

Table 2.3 Sources of Occupational Inhalant Allergens ... 17

Table 3.1 Common Environmental Allergens by Season in the Northern United States 25

Table 4.1 Differential Diagnosis of Rhinitis 28

Table 5.1 House-Dust Mite-Control Measures 40

Table 6.1 Currently Available Pharmacologic Agents for Treatment of Rhinitis 44

Table 6.2 Relative Efficacy of Drugs in Treatment of Allergic Rhinitis 45

Table 6.3 Available H_1-Antihistamines 46

Table 6.4 Factors to Be Considered Among the Second-Generation Antihistamines 51

Table 6.5 Over-the-Counter Decongestants 58

Table 6.6 Steroid Nasal Inhalers/Sprays 62

Table 6.7 Relative Topical Vasoconstrictor Potency 63

Table 6.8 Clinically Distinguishing Factors of Newer Intranasal Steroids 65

Table 6.9 Miscellaneous Agents for Rhinitis 71

Table 6.10 Ophthalmic Agents 75

Table 6.11 Risk to Fetus of Allergy and Asthma Medications During Pregnancy 76

Table 8.1 Theories Regarding the Link Between Rhinitis and Asthma 84

Table 9.1 Differential Diagnosis of Rhinosinusitis 92

Table 9.2 Classification of Adult Rhinosinusitis 93

Table 10.1 Prevalence of Cross-Resistance Between Penicillin and Various Antibiotic Classes Among Strains of Penicillin-Nonsusceptible Strains of *Streptococcus Pneumoniae* 103

Table 10.2 Antimicrobial Agents Stratified by Pharmacodynamic Profile Against *Streptococcus pneumoniae* and *Haemophilus influenzae* 104

Table 10.3 Mechanisms of Action of Commonly Used Antimicrobials for Community-Acquired Respiratory Tract Infections 106

Table 12.1 Antimicrobial Agents for Acute Bacterial Rhinosinusitis 118

Table 12.2 Recommended Antibiotic Therapy for Adults With ABRS 124

Table 12.3 Recommended Antibiotic Therapy for Children With ABRS 128

Table 13.1 Measures for Diagnosing Chronic Rhinosinusitis for Adult Clinical Care 136

FIGURES

Figure 3.1 Production of IgE Antibody and the Allergic Response 22

Figure 3.2 Summary of Proposed Mechanisms for Inflammation in Allergic Rhinitis 23

Figure 3.3 Early- and Late-Phase Allergic Response 24

Figure 4.1 Overlap of Serum IgE Levels in Allergic Disease 36

Figure 8.1 Summary of the Hypotheses Explaining the Links Between Rhinitis and Asthma 85

Figure 8.2 Allergic and Nonallergic Asthma 86

Figure 10.1 Schematic Drawing (Coronal View) of Nose and Paranasal Sinuses 96

Figure 10.2 Ranges of Prevalence of the Major Pathogens Associated With Acute Bacterial Rhinosinusitis in Adults 98

Figure 10.3 Microbiology of Acute Bacterial Rhinosinusitis in Children 99

Figure 10.4 Antibiotic Inactivation by β-Lactamases Such as Those of *Haemophilus influenzae* and *Moraxella catarrhalis* 100

Figure 10.5 Prevalence of Nonsusceptible Intermediate and Resistant *Streptococcus pneumoniae* to Penicillin 102

Figure 10.6 Prevalence of β-Lactamase Production by *Haemophilus influenzae* in the United States From 1997 to 2003 102

Figure 10.7 Major Antibiotic Targets of the Prokaryotic Cell 106

Figure 11.1 Plain Radiograph of Left Maxillary Air-Fluid Level 110

Figure 11.2 Simple Computed Tomography of Normal Paranasal Sinuses 111

Figure 11.3 Simple Computed Tomography of Deviated Septum 112

Figure 11.4 Simple Computed Tomography of Septal Spur 113

Figure 11.5 Simple Computed Tomography of Left Maxillary Polyp 114

Figure 11.6 Simple Computed Tomography of Bilateral Sinusitis 115

Figure 12.1 Sinus and Allergy Health Partnership—Recommended Antibiotic Therapy for Adults With ABRS 122

Figure 13.1 Computer-Aided Endoscopic Sinus Surgery 138

Figure 14.1 Coronal Computed Tomography Scan Demonstrating Bilateral Maxillary Sinus Opacification 143

Figure 14.2 Axial Computed Tomography Scan Demonstrating Left Ophthalmopathy 144

COLOR PLATES

Color Plate 1	View of Lateral Wall of Nose Demonstrating Relationships of Sinus Openings
Color Plate 2	Nasal Endoscopic Image of Right Lateral Nasal Wall
Color Plate 3	Nasal Examination and Culture
Color Plate 4	Radiograph Demonstrating Bilateral Air-Fluid Levels of Maxillary Sinuses
Color Plate 5	Plain Radiograph of Right Maxillary Opacification
Color Plate 6	Antrochoanal Polyp
Color Plate 7	Computed Tomography Scans of Various Degrees of Acute and Chronic Rhinosinusitis
Color Plate 8	Computed Tomography Scan Demonstrating Air-Fluid Levels
Color Plate 9	Computed Tomography Scan Demonstrating Air-Fluid Levels and Opacification
Color Plate 10	Nasal Endoscopic Examination Demonstrating Thick Nasal Secretions
Color Plate 11	Three Days After Initial Symptoms of Left Nasal Congestion and Left Facial Pain

1 Introduction

Rhinitis is defined as inflammation of the lining of the nose; rhinosinusitis, as inflammation of the lining of the paranasal sinuses due to any etiology. Both conditions are extremely common and affect individuals during productive years of childhood and young adulthood. Allergic rhinitis has been estimated to affect 40 million Americans, resulting in over 20 million physician visits each year. With about 10 million prescriptions written for nasal corticosteroids in the United States and about 1 billion prescriptions for antihistamines in 1995 worldwide, the direct treatment cost for chronic rhinitis is at least $3 billion in the United States. In addition, there is a significant indirect cost to days lost from the workplace as well as restriction from leisurely activities. A diagnosis of rhinitis or "allergic rhinitis" is typically based on an appropriate history and physical findings correlated with allergy skin testing or *in vitro* testing. A detailed environmental history to identify the presence of external triggers is also essential for both diagnosis and subsequent therapy.

Rhinosinusitis develops in approximately 30 million Americans each year, with an average of 4 days lost from work because of acute rhinosinusitis. Adult rhinosinusitis typically follows a viral upper respiratory infection. According to the National Ambulatory Medical Care Survey data, rhinosinusitis is the fifth most common diagnosis for which an antibiotic is prescribed. Rhinosinusitis accounted for 7% to 12% of all antibiotic prescriptions written from 1985 to 1992. In 1996, the primary diagnosis of rhinosinusitis led to expenditures of approximately $3.5 billion in the

United States. In general, a diagnosis of acute bacterial rhinosinusitis is made in adults or children when symptoms of a viral respiratory tract infection have not improved after 5 to 7 days. Plain film radiographs can be useful in the diagnosis of rhinosinusitis. A more definitive diagnosis is obtained from bacteriologic culture, which can be performed endoscopically or via sinus tap.

The goals of therapy for chronic rhinitis and rhinosinusitis include:

- Restoration of nasal patency and nasal function
- Control of nasal secretions
- Treatment of complications related to obstruction
- Prevention of recurrent symptoms.

This manual will review the pathogenesis, classification, differential diagnosis, and clinical evaluation, as well as overall management (nonpharmacologic and pharmacologic) of both rhinitis and rhinosinusitis. There will be emphasis on recent developments and advances. The section on rhinosinusitis reflects antimicrobial treatment guidelines issued by the Sinus and Allergy Health Partnership, a joint multidisciplinary effort.

2 Rhinitis: Definition, Classification, and Epidemiology

Rhinitis is defined as inflammation of the lining of the nose; rhinosinusitis, as inflammation of the nose and the lining of the paranasal sinuses. Both conditions may be acute or chronic. The cause may be infectious, immunologic, or nonimmunologic.

The common cold is the most common form of acute rhinitis. In addition to nasal symptoms, viral rhinitis is characterized by myalgia or sore throat and follows a predictable course to resolution within 10 days to 2 weeks. Viral respiratory infection may also cause self-limited acute infectious rhinosinusitis. The patient with a "summer cold" lasting a full month is likely to have allergic rhinitis. Allergic rhinitis may also occur in an acute form, such as on direct contact with a cat or during the peak of an offending pollen season.

A number of distinct disorders comprise the chronic rhinitis syndrome. The distinguishing features of these disorders are summarized in **Table 2.1**. Anatomic contribution to chronic nasal congestion must be considered in all forms of chronic rhinitis. Nasal septal deformity may be congenital or acquired. The middle turbinates may be wider than normal due to the congenital presence of an air cell in the turbinate (concha bullosa). Nasal polyps are inflammatory obstructions and are usually found in adults (except in cystic fibrosis). Adenoid hypertrophy may obstruct the nasal passages of children and adolescents.

TABLE 2.1 — Chronic Rhinitis Syndromes

	Allergic Rhinitis	Vasomotor Instability	NARES	Rhinitis Medicamentosa	Structural Rhinitis	Rhinosinusitis	Nasal Polyps
Cause or mechanisms	Allergens hyperreactivity	Vascular	Unknown	Medication abnormalities	Septal	Infection	Inflammation
Sneezing and pruritus	Moderate	Absent	Marked	Absent	Absent	Absent	Absent
Rhinorrhea	Moderate	Questionable	Marked	Absent	Absent	Purulent	Slight
Congestion	Mild	Marked	Questionable	Moderate	Moderate	Mild	Marked
Postnasal drainage	Slight	Marked	Questionable	Absent	Absent	Moderate	Mild
Seasonal variation	Seasonal or perennial	Perennial	Perennial	Perennial	Perennial	Perennial	Perennial
Eosinophils in nasal secretion	Slight	Absent	Slight	Absent	Absent	Absent	Slight
Skin test results	Positive	Negative	Negative	Negative	Negative	Negative	Negative
Total IgE	Increased	Normal	Normal	Normal	Normal	Normal	Normal

Age at onset	Childhood	Adults	All ages	Adults	All ages	All ages	Adults
Associated factors	Family history, pale mucosa	Pregnancy, thyroid dis-order	Pale mucosa	Use of topical decongestants, antihypertensives	Unilateral with obstruction; his-tory of nasal trauma	Associated upper respira-tory infection	Aspirin sensitivity
Treatment	Topical steroids, environmental control, immuno-therapy	Decongestant, nasal saline, exercise	Topical steroids	Stop medication	Surgery	Antibiotics	Topical steroids, surgery

Abbreviations: IgE, immunoglobulin E; NARES, nonallergic rhinitis with eosinophilia syndrome.

Modified from: Slavin RG. *Ann Allergy*. 1982;49:123.

Allergic Rhinitis

Allergic rhinitis is the most common allergic disease, occurring in 20 to 30 million people in the United States, with a prevalence in 10% to 30% of the adult population and up to 40% in children. It is defined as acute and chronic nasal inflammation triggered by specific immunoglobulin (IgE)-mediated reactions to inhalant allergens and associated with eosinophils in the nasal mucosa.

Most patients with allergic rhinitis have multiple inhalant sensitivities; pure ragweed allergy is the exception rather than the rule.

Vasomotor Rhinitis

Some patients have a hyperreactive nose, responding in an exaggerated fashion to nonspecific irritants without allergic sensitization. These stimuli may include:

- Smoke
- Air pollution
- Odors
- Occupational irritants and allergens (**Table 2.2** and **Table 2.3**).

These patients lack the itchy, watery eyes usually found along with an itchy, watery nose in allergic rhinitis/conjunctivitis. In fact, the absence of conjunctivitis casts doubt on a diagnosis of allergic rhinitis.

Nonallergic Rhinitis With Eosinophilia Syndrome

In this condition, as in the allergic form, eosinophils are found in nasal secretions, but the patient does not have allergies. A similar observation is frequently

TABLE 2.2 — Occupational Irritants

- Cleaning agents
- Cooking odors
- Cosmetic odors
- Detergents
- Exhaust fumes
- Tobacco smoke
- Paint fumes
- Solvents
- Ammonia
- Cold air
- Formaldehyde
- Hair sprays
- Acids
- Chlorine

Adapted from: Slavin RG. *Allergy and Asthma Proceedings.* 1998;19:277-284.

TABLE 2.3 — Sources of Occupational Inhalant Allergens

- Animals
- Grains
- Coffee beans
- Wood dusts
- Latex
- Enzymes
- Acid anhydrides
- Colophony
- Cotton fibers
- Green tea
- Papain
- Platinum salts
- Toluene diisocyanate

Adapted from: Slavin RG. *Allergy and Asthma Proceedings.* 1998;19:277-284.

made in asthma; an abundance of eosinophils are found in the bronchial secretions even though the patient does not have allergies.

Rhinitis Medicamentosa

Physicians must be aware that patients may affect their nasal condition by chronic use of decongestant sprays. Intermittent rhinitis may become constant (rhinitis medicamentosa) due to the rebound swelling between frequent doses of the sprays.

Severe nasal congestion may also be associated with pregnancy. Birth control pills (pseudopregnancy) occasionally cause nasal congestion. Hypothyroid patients may also experience nasal congestion.

Gustatory Rhinitis

Rhinorrhea occurring during and after meals, usually seen in patients over age 60, is referred to as gustatory rhinitis. These patients may suspect food allergy, but food skin tests are negative and there is no preceding history of allergic rhinitis. The disorder seems to be due to nasal serous gland secretion at a time when there should be gastrointestinal gland secretion.

Asthma and Allergic Rhinitis

Disorders involving the nasal passages or the sinus cavities frequently accompany the symptoms of asthma. There is a substantial overlap between patients with asthma, rhinitis, and nasal polyposis. As many as 50% to 80% of patients with asthma have rhinitis symptoms, whereas 10% to 15% of those with perennial rhinitis have asthmatic symptoms. Methacholine responsiveness in the asthmatic range is seen in a significant number of patients with no overt history of asthma.

Nasal Polyps

According to a study of 5,000 patients with asthma and/or allergic rhinitis, 17% of asthmatics had nasal polyps, whereas 70% of patients with nasal polyps had asthma. Nasal polyps associated with rhinitis and asthma are seen primarily in patients who are over age 40. Asthmatic aspirin sensitivity is seen in >30% of asthmatic patients with nasal polyps. Although aspirin sensitivity is not mediated by immunoglobulin E (IgE), ingestion of aspirin may trigger severe asthma. Nasal polyps are at least twice as prevalent in patients with rhinitis and in asthma patients who have negative skin tests as in those with positive skin tests. The exact etiology of nasal polyposis is unclear, but it seems to be related to an inflammation of the nasal mucosa. This suggests that nasal polyps are probably a manifestation not of allergy, but of the underlying eosinophilic hypertrophic rhinosinusitis that accompanies severe asthma and rhinitis. Medications capable of shrinking polyps include topical and systemic corticosteroids. A high incidence of radiographic sinus abnormalities are seen in patients with asthma, perhaps >50%.

3 Rhinitis: Pathogenesis

3

The essential components of allergic reactions include:

- Allergens
- Immunoglobulin E (IgE) antibodies
- Mast cells
- Eosinophils.

In allergic rhinitis, a complex inflammatory cascade results in the following pathophysiologic hallmarks in the nasal mucosa and submucosa:

- Vasodilatation and edema formation
- Engorgement of mucous glands and goblet cells
- Infiltration of the mucosa and submucosa with eosinophils.

Inhaled allergens penetrate mucosal barriers, such as the nasal mucosa, and are processed by an antigen-presenting cell, such as the macrophage (**Figure 3.1**). Lymphokines secreted by this interaction stimulate activation of the T helper 2 (T_{H2}) cell and causes the B cell to switch to a specific IgE-producing plasma cell. IgE antibody then binds to high-affinity receptors on mast cells as well as to receptors on eosinophils. When sensitized mast cells and eosinophils encounter the surface inhaled allergen, degranulation occurs and symptoms of rhinitis develop because of the chemical mediators released by the mast cell and eosinophil. **Figure 3.1** also depicts the functions of IgE (thin arrows) and interleukin-4 (IL-4) (thick arrows) in the allergic response. IL-4 induces T-cell activation and differentiation to T_{H2} cells and promotes the development of B cells into IgE-producing cells.

FIGURE 3.1 — Production of IgE Antibody and the Allergic Response

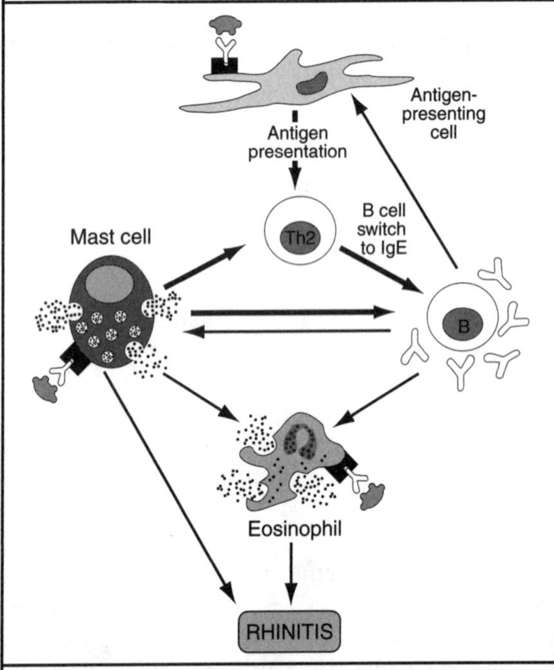

Abbreviations: B, B cell; IgE, immunoglobulin E; IL-4, interleukin 4; Th, T helper [lymphocyte].

IL-4 (thick arrow); IgE (thin arrow).

Holgate ST, Church MK, Lichtenstein LM. *Allergy*. 2nd ed. Philadelphia, Pa: Mosby International Ltd; 2001:243.

Figure 3.2 depicts a summary of proposed mechanisms for inflammation in allergic rhinitis. The isotype switch from B-lymphocyte production of immunoglobulin M (IgM) to production of IgE is promoted by IL-4, a T_{H2} interleukin cytokine. IL-5, another T_{H2} cytokine, stimulates eosinophil production. Interleukins 3, 4, and 10 stimulate growth of mast cells. Thus the antibodies and cells needed for the allergic

FIGURE 3.2 — Summary of Proposed Mechanisms for Inflammation in Allergic Rhinitis

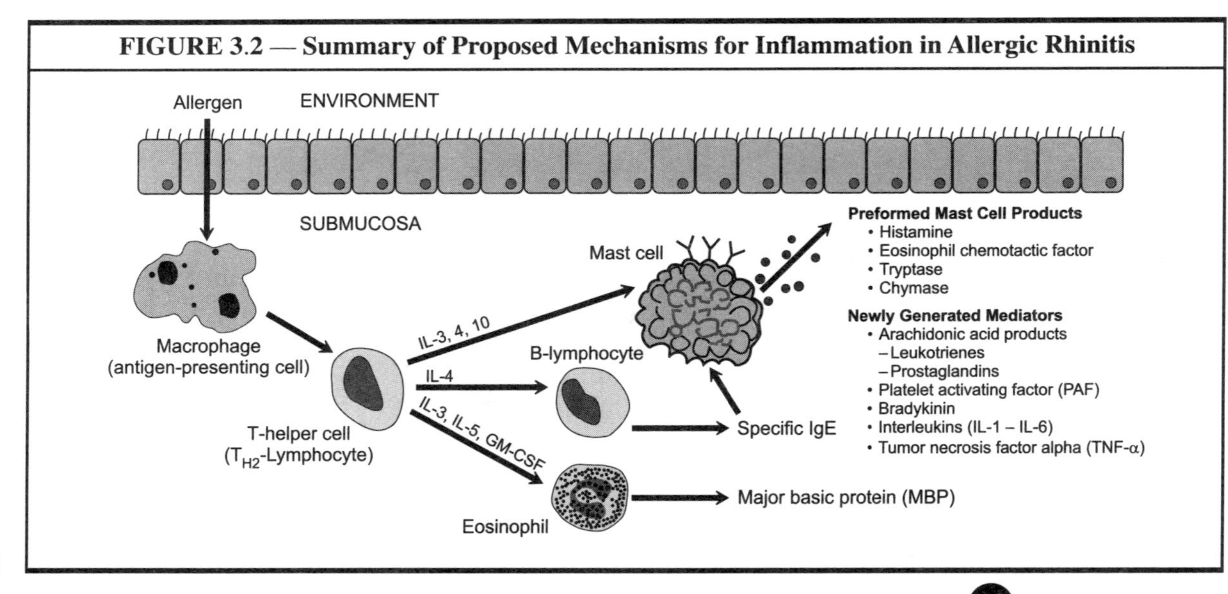

3

response are promoted by the cytokines of the T_{H2} lymphocytes. Specific IgE binds to high-affinity receptors on the mast-cell surface (**Figure 3.3**).

Bridging of two mast-cell–bound IgE molecules by allergen initiates mast-cell degranulation and subsequent secretion of a variety of chemical mediators. Histamine, a preformed mediator, is released early, followed by newly formed mediators.

FIGURE 3.3 — Early- and Late-Phase Allergic Response

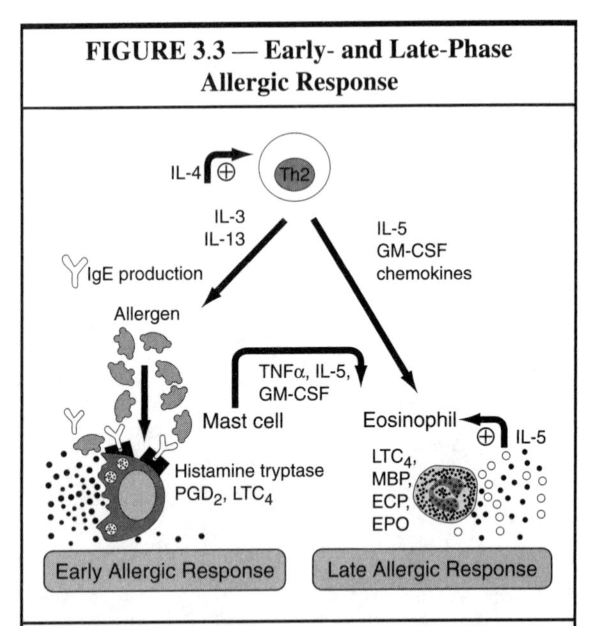

Abbreviations: EPO; eosinophil peroxidase; GM-CSF, granulocyte-macrophage colony-stimulating factor; IgE; immunoglobulin E; IL, interleukin; LTC_4, leukotriene C_4; MBP, eosinophil cationic protein; PGD, prostaglandin D; Th, T helper [lymphocyte]; TNF-α, tumor necrosis factor alpha.

Inflammatory cells, cytokines, and chemokines in early- and late-phase allegic responses.

Holgate ST, Church MK, Lichtenstein LM. *Allergy*. 2nd ed. Philadelphia, Pa: Mosby International Ltd; 2001:385.

Nasal itching is triggered by histamine and prostaglandins; sneezing and rhinorrhea, by histamine and leukotrienes; and nasal congestion is caused by histamine, kinins, leukotrienes, and tumor necrosis factor alpha (TNF-α). The role of antihistamines and topical corticosteroids, which inhibit the production of prostaglandins and leukotrienes in the symptomatic treatment of allergic rhinitis, is well justified; but many mediators are involved, and the future may call for more specific antimediator therapies. Part of the appeal of immunotherapy is that the allergic response to environmental allergens is blunted, and the release of chemical mediators is reduced after allergen exposure. **Table 3.1** is a list of common environmental allergies by season in the northern United States.

The autonomic nervous system also makes a significant contribution to the pathogenesis of rhinitis. Nasal patency is greatly influenced by the sympathetic

TABLE 3.1 — Common Environmental Allergens by Season in the Northern United States

Season	Allergen
Early spring (February-May)	Tree pollens (elm, oak, hickory, maple)
Late spring (May-June)	Grasses (rye varieties)
Summer (July-August)	Ground or outdoor molds (*Alternaria*, *Fusarium*, *Cladosporium*)
Fall (mid-August–October)	Ragweed (plus cocklebur, lamb's-quarter, pigweed, plantain)
Winter (November-February) and all year	Dust mites, animal emanations, cockroaches, molds (*Aspergillus*, *Alternaria*, *Penicillium*)

Kaliner M et al. *JAMA*. 1992;268:2808.

control of vascular tone. Rhinorrhea is under parasympathetic control. The peptide neurotransmitter (substance P) released from neurons may cause mast-cell degranulation as well as directly affect rhinorrhea and nasal congestion.

Many atopic individuals have a biphasic response to allergen challenge; this is known as an early- and late-phase response. The inflammatory cells, cytokines, and chemokines are illustrated in **Figure 3.2**. The immediate or early response occurs within several minutes and the symptoms are itching, sneezing, and rhinorrhea, which are mediated primarily by histamine when the mast cell degranulates. Additional mast-cell mediators, such as TNF-α, IL-5, and granulocyte-macrophage colony-stimulating factor (GM-CSF), have proinflammatory effects and can augment eosinophil growth and activation. Activated eosinophils are characteristic of the late allergic response and are also affected by T_{H2} mediators (IL-5, GM-CSF). The cellular infiltrate during the late phase also includes neutrophils and mononuclear cells. Nasal congestion is the predominant clinical symptom seen with late-phase inflammatory allergic response, which occurs several hours after the initial phase. Corticosteroids, cromolyn sodium, and immunotherapy can reduce severity of the congestion. Some of the second-generation antihistamines, such as azelastine, cetirizine, and loratadine, also appear to possess anti-inflammatory properties.

4 Rhinitis: Diagnosis

Patients may not realize that not all chronic rhinitis is the result of allergy and that both allergic and nonallergic factors may contribute to their nasal symptoms (**Table 4.1**). For example, structural obstruction of the nasal passages must be considered in all chronic rhinitis patients. Nasal septal deformity and nasal polyps in adults are the two most common obstructive factors contributing to chronic nasal symptoms. Nasal obstruction may be caused by adenoid hypertrophy in children and young adults. Rarely, malignant tumors or granulomatous disease may cause chronic rhinitis or obstruction. These illnesses are associated with constant symptoms, whereas allergic rhinitis is generally intermittent.

In patients who are always unable to breathe freely through the nose, an anatomic factor is suspect, whereas the intermittent ability to do so discounts the primary role of nasal obstruction. Fluctuations in obstruction are caused by soft tissue changes since bone and cartilage cannot change shape from day to day.

Questions that should be asked of all patients with a history of rhinitis include:

- Is your sleep disturbed by nasal congestion? (This is a major quality-of-life factor and may reflect unsuspected sleep apnea.)
- Have you lost your sense of smell/taste? (If so, this problem deserves aggressive investigation, including rhinoscopy and/or computed tomography of sinuses.)
- Do you have cough, wheezing, or shortness of breath? (Asthma frequently presents in patients with chronic rhinitis or sinusitis.)

TABLE 4.1 — Differential Diagnosis of Rhinitis
Allergic • Seasonal (hay fever, rose fever) • Perennial • Vasomotor • Perennial nonallergic
Nonallergic Rhinitis With Eosinophils (NARES)
Infectious
Secondary Rhinitis • Rhinitis medicamentosa • Pregnancy • Ciliary dyskinesia • Other local conditions – Polyps – Septal deviation – Tumor – Wegener's granulomatosis – Foreign body
Modified from: Kaliner M et al. *JAMA*. 1992;268:2811.

Questions that may be helpful in leading the clinician toward or away from a diagnosis of allergic rhinitis include:

- Does your nose itch? (Nasal itching and sneezing are nearly always present.)
- Do your eyes itch? (Some allergic conjunctivitis is nearly always present.)
- Are your symptoms worse in pollen season or around animals? ("Yes" is strongly suggestive of allergy.)

Allergic rhinitis usually presents for the first time in a young person. In >70% of patients, symptoms develop before age 30, and in most patients, subside by age 50. Thus the onset of nasal symptoms after age 50 rarely has an allergic basis. Nasal polyps are a common cause of new, persistent nasal congestion in middle age and later years; they are discussed in other chapters of this monograph. A detailed environmental history to elicit the presence of external triggers is helpful both for diagnosis and for subsequent avoidance therapy.

Symptoms and Signs

Typical symptoms include:

- Sneezing
- Nasal pruritus
- Rhinorrhea with associated postnasal drip
- Nasal congestion
- Itching and watering of the eyes
- Itching of the pharynx.

Severe symptoms at peak season may interfere with sleep and cause fatigue. Loss of appetite may occur secondary to loss of the sense of smell. Headache and pain are not usually primary allergic symptoms; recurrent chronic headache in the absence of sinusitis probably represents a second diagnosis, such as tension or vascular headache.

Patients may have a history of childhood eczema in the atopic dermatitis pattern of antecubital and popliteal distribution. First-degree relatives often have allergic rhinitis or asthma. A child whose parent has allergic rhinitis has a 30% chance of having it as well, and if both parents are affected, the chance rises to the range of 60%.

Consistent flare of symptoms around animals strongly suggests an allergic cause. The non–pet owner who is allergic to animal dander has respiratory symptoms within minutes of contact with an animal or upon entering the house in which it lives. Allergic patients may even react to animal dander on the clothes of pet owners outside their homes. Prolonged daily exposure and persistence of animal allergens on clothes result in persistence of symptoms in allergic pet owners even away from home.

Seasonal Pollen Counts

Interpretation of the seasonal variation in symptoms is complex. Pollen seasons vary according to geographic location:

- Northeast and Midwest tree pollen season begins in March, extends into June, with trees pollinating in sequence, but many overlapping: willow and cottonwood in early spring; then maple, which peaks by mid-April; followed by birch in early May and oak in late May.
- Midwest grass pollen reaches higher concentrations than in the Northeast, causing a significant allergic problem in June and July. Ragweed pollen dominates from mid-August to late September.
- Southeast tree pollen emerges as early as mid-January.
- In the South, northern grasses (timothy, blue grass, orchard grass, rye grass, and red top) are joined by Bermuda grass, whose antigens are not cross-reactive with the northern grasses. In southern Florida, grass may pollinate year-round.
- On the West Coast, the olive is a major pollinating tree; much of this area is free of ragweed.

In perennial allergic rhinitis, symptoms fluctuate in severity but recur throughout the year. Except in the deep South, pollen disappears from the air for at least a month or two in the winter. Perennial allergic rhinitis is more dependent than seasonal rhinitis on skin testing to establish the diagnosis.

Indoor allergens, primarily house-dust mites and animal dander, are present all year. Some patients with mite sensitivity may notice a flair of symptoms when dusting or using a vacuum cleaner.

Mold Spore Counts

The role of molds in allergic disease is not well understood. Mold spore counts may exceed pollen counts. Mold spores are in the air to some extent any time the ground is not covered by snow. *Alternaria* and *Cladosporium* are among the most common outdoor mold spores found in the air. Mold spores may contribute to allergic rhinitis during the warm months of the year.

A few patients will present with a consistent summer pattern of symptoms, yet have negative pollen and mold skin tests. Air temperature, humidity, and air pollution may also contribute to a seasonal pattern of symptoms.

Medication History

The clinical history of a patient with chronic rhinitis always includes a history of medications. Chronic (even once daily) use of decongestant sprays (oxymetazoline or phenylephrine) may induce rebound nasal congestion. Rhinitis may also be caused by:

- Blood pressure medications (angiotensin-converting enzyme inhibitors, reserpine, guanethidine, phentolamine, methyldopa, prazosin, and β-blockers)
- Pregnancy
- Birth control pills
- Foods (rare without gastrointestinal and/or cutaneous evidence of allergic reaction)
- Food ingestion
- Alcohol (due to vasoactive chemicals).

Physical Examination

The allergic status of an individual is determined by the allergy history and skin testing, not by examination of the nose. Anterior nasal examination may detect the presence of anatomic factors, such as septal deviation or nasal polyps. The nasal speculum offers a view of the anterior nasal passages, which, in patients with chronic nasal obstruction, may be limited to little more than the nasal vestibule.

Nasal endoscopic evaluation using a flexible or rigid endoscope provides the best means of physical diagnosis of anatomic obstruction of the nasal passages, which is particularly important in patients with chronic rhinosinusitis. Nasal patency may be estimated by asking the patient to inhale through the nose while gently occluding one nasal passage with pressure on the alar cartilage. Given constant obstruction on one or both sides, an anatomic basis must be sought. Nasal endoscopy may reveal polyps, severe septal deviation, massive adenoids, or intranasal neoplasms.

Examination of the nose begins with description of the shape of the nasal septum and its contribution to nasal obstruction, but the presence of ulcerations or perforations should be sought and noted. Examination of the nose during uncomplicated allergic rhinitis typically shows edematous, pale, bluish nasal turbinates covered with thin, clear secretions. These inflammatory changes may obstruct the nasal airway and partially block the ostia ventilating the sinuses, leading to the complication of rhinosinusitis.

A patient with allergic rhinitis may have a red mucosa resulting from complications due to:

- Viral infection
- Smoking
- Decongestant spray abuse.

Allergic obstruction of the nose is inherently temporary; when the allergen is gone, the rhinitis improves. Moreover, in allergic rhinitis, the nasal discharge is usually watery and clear, whereas viral rhinitis is characterized by a more tenacious white, yellow, or green discharge. If a purulent discharge is directly observed streaming from a sinus ostium or from the middle meatus lateral to the middle turbinate, the diagnosis of infectious rhinosinusitis may be established by physical examination. Rhinoscopy may be necessary to make this observation.

A pale, edematous mucosa may also be seen in nonallergic rhinitis with eosinophilia syndrome (NARES). The peripheral eosinophil count may be elevated in allergic rhinitis or asthma, but eosinophilia is also closely correlated with the extent of sinus disease, even in the absence of atopy.

Laboratory and Skin Tests

In allergic rhinitis or asthma, the peripheral eosinophil count may be elevated, but this is nonspecific. Eosinophils may predominate in allergic rhinitis and asthma, whereas in infectious rhinitis, a smear of nasal secretions or nasal scraping typically shows polymorphonuclear leukocytes.

Diagnosis of allergic rhinitis usually requires detection of specific immunoglobulin (IgE) to environmental allergens by immunoassay of a blood sample or by skin testing. However, skin testing is the method of choice when the skin is suitable (without generalized urticaria or eczema); it has greater sensitivity and permits less expensive testing for a larger number of allergens.

To avoid false-negative skin tests, both histamine $(H)_1$- and H_2-blockers must be discontinued at least 2 days beforehand. Antihistamines, such as hydroxyzine and astemizole, may need to be discontinued for 1 to 4 weeks. Oral and topical corticosteroids do not interfere with immediate hypersensitivity skin testing, and asthma medications need not be stopped. In all patients, control-negative (diluent) and control-positive (histamine) skin tests should be applied and compared to the allergen skin tests.

Allergy skin testing materials consist of simple aqueous extracts of proteins from:

- Pollens
- Molds
- Dust mites and mite fecal pellets
- Animal danders
- Foods.

Food extracts are used for diagnosis only, whereas inhalant extracts are used for both skin testing and immunotherapy.

A negative intradermal skin test with a normal positive control essentially rules out the presence of specific IgE to the allergen tested. Although the negative test does not rule out other mechanisms of reaction to an inhaled or ingested substance, immunotherapy need not be considered in the absence of a positive test. On the other hand, the positive skin test proves the potential for allergic reaction but does not prove that an allergic mechanism is responsible for the patient's illness. Positive skin tests must be correlated with the patient's clinical history to reach a final diagnosis of allergic rhinitis.

Allergy skin testing usually starts with prick or puncture testing. Comprehensive testing includes individual extracts from locally important trees, grasses, and weeds, as well as cats, dogs, dust mites, and molds. A drop of each extract is placed on the skin of the back or arm, and a variety of devices are used to puncture or prick the skin through the drop, forcing a minute amount of extract into the skin. If specific IgE is present for the antigens tested, wheal and flare reactions develop at the site(s) within 15 minutes. Once the test is read, the excess extract is wiped off.

Some physicians follow negative prick tests with intradermal injection of extracts that are at least 25 times more dilute than those used in prick testing. Despite the dilution, the intradermal test is more sensitive than the prick test.

■ Skin Test Extracts

Some extracts have been standardized for allergenic potency, with the concentration expressed in allergy units (AU) or biologic allergy units (BAU) per cubic centimeter; the higher the AU or BAU per cc, the more potent the extract. Some extracts are labeled according to the older, less accurate protein nitrogen units and some, according to the weight-by-volume method: for example, a 1:50 ragweed extract consists of the proteins extracted from 1 g of ragweed pollen in 50 cc of diluent. The higher the denominator, the more dilute and less potent the extract. All grass extracts for sale in the United States are now in BAU/cc. Ragweed is standardized by allergen content, but is still sold in weight/volume dilution. Immunotherapy for a variety of aeroallergens may involve one or more extract with different units of potency. Preparation of extracts should be in the hands of an experienced allergist.

■ Blood Tests

Radioallergosorbent (RAST) or enzyme-linked immunosorbent assay (ELISA) for human IgE to specific allergens are *in vitro* tests that can be run on a serum sample if the skin cannot be used for testing. The main advantage of the *in vitro* assay is its safety; the patient is not exposed to the test allergen, obviating the risk of systemic allergic reaction (**Figure 4.1**). A disadvantage is the need to run a separate test for

FIGURE 4.1 — Overlap of Serum IgE Levels in Allergic Disease

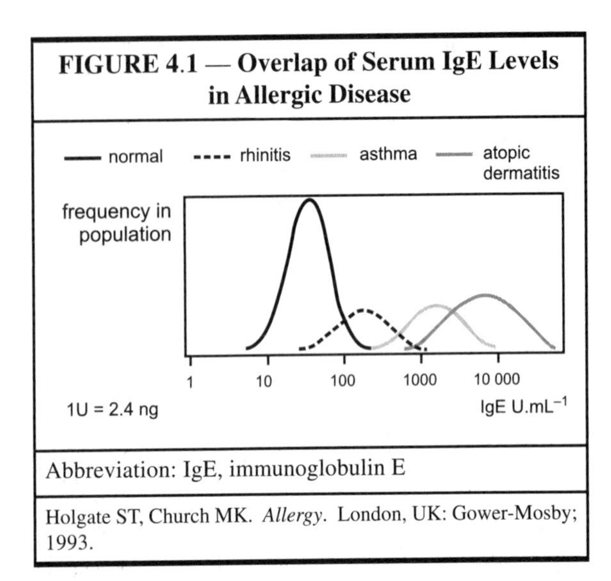

Abbreviation: IgE, immunoglobulin E

Holgate ST, Church MK. *Allergy*. London, UK: Gower-Mosby; 1993.

each allergen tested, and the cost is a direct multiple of number of tests run. Skin tests, on the other hand, can involve multiple allergens with little additional cost. Furthermore, the results of skin testing are known in 15 minutes, whereas those of *in vitro* testing are not known for hours or days.

However, *in vitro* tests are still less sensitive than skin testing, which remains the method of choice for allergy specialists. For *in vitro* as well as skin testing, positive test results must be considered in light of the clinical history. Allergy skin tests for ragweed remain positive long after the clinical allergic rhinitis has ceased to recur.

Complications of Rhinitis

Complications of chronic inflammation of the nasal passages include:

- Otitis media
- Rhinosinusitis.

Otitis media is more common in children, while acute rhinosinusitis is more common in adults.

■ Otitis Media

Nasal mucosal edema and excess secretions may obstruct the eustachian tube, resulting in otitis media. Examination may show a retracted tympanic membrane with decreased motion or no motion on pneumatic otoscopy. Tympanometry can document the loss of normal eardrum movement. Audiometry can document a conductive hearing loss. Otitis media may require antibiotic therapy. If middle ear pressure cannot be equalized by medical means, placement of ventilating tubes through the eardrums may be considered to alleviate the middle ear effusion and improve the associated conductive hearing loss.

Guidelines for Allergic Rhinitis

There are two commonly referred-to guidelines for allergic rhinitis. The first document is *Diagnosis and Management of Rhinitis: Parameter Documents of the Joint Task Force on Practice Parameters in Allergy, Asthma, and Immunology*. It is a joint effort from the American College of Allergy, Asthma, and Immunology and the American Academy of Allergy, Asthma, and Immunology. These practice parameters from 1998 classify the various types of rhinitis and discuss management and complications of rhinitis. They also review allergen immunotherapy and additional considerations in patient subsets, such as children, the elderly, and pregnant women. More recently in 2003, the Joint Task Force on Practice Parameters reconvened to develop a symptom-severity assessment for allergic rhinitis. This document includes measurements for nasal symptom severity, non-nasal symptom severity, global severity, quality-of-life issues, and the impact of medications.

The second set of guidelines is commonly referred to as ARIA—*Allergic Rhinitis and Its Impact on Asthma*. The ARIA report was published in November 2001 and developed in collaboration with the World Health Organization. Leaders of the ARIA group are Jean Bousquet and Paul van Cauwenberge. This document is a comprehensive review of rhinitis and the epidemiology, genetics, and mechanisms causing symptoms of rhinitis. The assessment of severity of rhinitis is discussed and guidance on management based on the symptom severity is provided. The ARIA guidelines have proposed a new subdivision of allergic rhinitis with intermittent and persistent definitions, as well as classifying allergic rhinitis as mild or moderate/severe. The ARIA report also provides a stepwise approach to the use of medications recommended in the treatment of allergic rhinitis. Finally, the ARIA report emphasizes that allergic rhinitis is a major chronic respiratory disease and that patients with persistent allergic rhinitis should also be evaluated for asthma.

5 Rhinitis: Nonpharmacologic Therapy

The general goals of therapy for chronic rhinitis syndrome include:

- Restoration of nasal patency
- Control of nasal secretions
- Treatment of complications such as bacterial infection.

There are three specific approaches to management:

- Avoidance of the responsible allergens
- Pharmacotherapy (see Chapter 6, *Rhinitis: Pharmacologic Therapy*):
  - Antihistamines
  - Decongestants
  - Intranasal corticosteroids
  - Cromolyn sodium
  - Anticholinergics
  - Ocular therapy.
- Immunotherapy by subcutaneous injection of increasing quantities of allergen (in selected patients) (see Chapter 7, *Rhinitis: Immunotherapy*).

Avoidance of Responsible Allergens

Allergy skin testing is essential for management of chronic rhinitis if immunotherapy is being considered. The results of skin tests are helpful in establishment of a diagnosis and in treatment, even when immunotherapy is not being considered. The skin test results guide recommendations concerning any environmental control that may be needed.

In seasonal rhinitis, the skin tests usually confirm pollen sensitivity. Outdoor pollen cannot be avoided, but the indoor pollen count can be greatly reduced by use of air-conditioning, thus permitting the windows to be closed during pollen season. Air-conditioning should also be used in the car during pollen season. Patients with pollen or mold allergy should not mow the grass or rake leaves.

In year-round, chronic rhinitis, house-dust mite allergens and animal dander allergens may be contributing factors. House-dust mite control measures are extensive (**Table 5.1**). There are some recent updates in the medical literature regarding house-dust mite avoidance measures. Sheikh and Hurwitz performed a search to assess the benefits of mite avoidance measures in the treatment of allergic rhinitis. The authors commented on only four studies that fulfilled the criteria of a randomized controlled trial. Different means of

TABLE 5.1 — House-Dust Mite–Control Measures
Essential • Encase the mattress in a mite barrier cover • Encase the pillow in a mite barrier cover • Wash the bedding in water of 130° F weekly • Avoid sleeping or lying on upholstered furniture • Remove carpets that are laid on concrete
Desirable • Reduce indoor humidity to <50% • Remove carpets from the bedroom • Use chemical agents to kill mites or to alter the mite antigens in the house
National Asthma Education Program: expert panel report. *Guidelines for the Diagnosis and Management of Asthma.* Bethesda, Md: National Institutes of Health; 1991:66.

avoidance measures were employed in the studies and included the use of:

- Acaricides
- High-efficiency particulate air (HEPA) filters
- Bedroom environmental-control program that used mite-proof mattress covers.

The authors concluded that there were few studies of high methodologic quality and that while interventions to decrease mite exposure in the home may be of benefit, actual efficacy has been difficult to ascertain.

Since the Sheikh and Hurwitz article from 1998, a more recent study by Terreehorst and colleagues has been published in the *New England Journal of Medicine* in 2003. This study was a randomized, double-blind, placebo-controlled trial that involved three medical centers and evaluated 232 patients with allergic rhinitis. Patients were randomized to receive impermeable or nonimpermeable covers for the beds. The results showed that impermeable covers do significantly reduce mite proteins, but that there was no significant outcome on clinical measures (patient-measured disease severity, daily nasal-symptom score, nasal allergen–provocation score).

Another recent study evaluating environmental control measures for children with asthma employed several control measures. This study was a large (937 children) multicenter, randomized, controlled trial that utilized education and implementation of allergen-impermeable covers, HEPA filter vacuum cleaners, HEPA air purifiers, and professional pest control for cockroaches. These measures were to decrease both allergen and tobacco smoke exposures and were maintained for 1 year. The authors found that these interventions reduced reported asthma symptom days and unscheduled visits to the emergency room or to clinics. It was concluded that multiple control measures can reduce morbidity in inner city children with allergic asthma.

It is therefore recommended to atopic patients that environmental control measures need to be instituted in the home to decrease both indoor and outdoor allergens. A comprehensive environmental control program would then be expected to be beneficial in controlling and minimizing symptoms of allergic rhinoconjunctivitis.

6 Rhinitis: Pharmacologic Therapy

Pharmacologic agents available for the treatment of rhinitis include:

- Oral antihistamines
- Intranasal antihistamines
- Intranasal corticosteroids
- Intranasal cromolyn sodium
- Intranasal anticholinergics
- Decongestants
- Leukotriene modifiers.

Table 6.1 lists the available agents by drug class. Their relative efficacy in controlling the major symptoms of rhinitis is indicated in **Table 6.2**.

6

Oral Antihistamines

Histamine remains an important mediator of symptoms in allergic rhinitis and conjunctivitis, and histamine-receptor antagonists are widely prescribed for the symptomatic management of allergic rhinitis. These agents are effective in relieving nasal itching, rhinorrhea, and sneezing, but are less effective in controlling nasal congestion. Antihistamines work by preventing the binding of histamine in the target tissue; they do not reverse any action already taken by histamine. Thus they are most effective when taken daily during a period of allergen exposure. In addition to competitively blocking the binding of histamine by histamine-1 (H_1) receptors, some of the agents in this class also block the release of histamine and perhaps other mediators from mast cells. In addition, recent

TABLE 6.1 — Currently Available Pharmacologic Agents for Treatment of Rhinitis
Antihistamines (Table 6.3) • First generation • Second generation • Intranasal antihistamines
Inhaled Sympathomimetics (Table 6.5) • *Short-acting*: – Epinephrine – Naphazoline – Phenylephrine – Tetrahydrozoline • *Long-acting*: – Oxymetazoline – Xylometazoline
Oral Sympathomimetics • Pseudoephedrine
Steroid Nasal Inhalers (Table 6.6) • Beclomethasone dipropionate • Budesonide • Dexamethasone sodium phosphate • Flunisolide • Fluticasone • Mometasone • Triamcinolone acetonide
Cromoglycates • Cromolyn sodium solution
Anticholinergics • Ipratropium bromide
Leukotrienes • Montelukast
Hybrid Nasal Sprays

TABLE 6.2 — Relative Efficacy of Drugs in Treatment of Allergic Rhinitis			
Drug	**Symptoms**		
	Sneezing	**Congestion**	**Secretions**
Anticholinergic	–	–	++
Antihistamine	++	–	+
Cromolyn sodium	+	+	+
Decongestant	–	++	–
Leukotriene	+	+	+
Nasal steroid	++	++	++

work suggests that antihistamines may also block the influx of eosinophils following allergen challenge.

Antihistamines can be broadly classified as:

- First generation (sedating):
  - Brompheniramine
  - Chlorpheniramine
  - Diphenhydramine
  - Hydroxyzine
- Second generation (non- or mildly sedating):
  - Cetirizine (Zyrtec)
  - Desloratadine (Clarinex)
  - Fexofenadine (Allegra)
  - Loratadine (Claritin).

See **Table 6.3** for list of available H_1-receptor antagonists.

A number of placebo-controlled, prospective studies have clearly shown that both first- and second-generation antihistamines are effective in reducing the symptoms of allergic rhinitis except for congestion. One of the advantages of oral antihistamines is that they help control ocular as well as nasal itching. Their lack of influence on nasal congestion leads the phar-

TABLE 6.3 — Available H_1-Antihistamines

Class/Generic Name	Trade Name	Dosage (Adult)	Dosage (Children ≤12 years)
FIRST-GENERATION ANTIHISTAMINES			
Alkylamines			
Brompheniramine maleate	Dimetane, others*	4 mg, 3-4 times/d	0.4 mg/kg, in 3-4 divided doses/d
Chlorpheniramine maleate	Chlor-Trimeton, others*	4 mg, 3-4 times/d	<2 y, 1.25 mg, 2-3 times daily; 0.4 mg/kg in 3-4 divided doses/d
Ethanolamine			
Diphenhydramine HCl	Benadryl*	25-50 mg, 3-4 times/d	5 mg/kg, in 3-4 divided doses/d
Phenothiazines			
Promethazine HCl	Phenergan[†]	25 mg hs, or 12.5 bid before meals and hs	≥2 years: 25 mg hs, or 6.25-12.5 mg tid
Piperazines			
Azatadine maleate	Optimine[†]	1-2 mg, 2 times/d	No recommendation given for children
	Trinalin[†]	1 mg bid	Not intended for use in children >12 years
Hydroxyzine HCl	Atarax[†]	25 mg tid or qid	<6 years: 50 mg/d in divided doses; ≥6 years: 50-100 mg/d in divided doses
	Vistaril[†]	25 mg tid or qid	<6 years: 50 mg/d in divided doses; >6 years: 50-100 mg/d in divided doses

Miscellaneous			
Clemastine fumarate	Tavist 1*, Tavist D*, Tavist†	1.34 mg, 2.68 mg, 2 times/d	No recommendation given for children
Cyproheptadine HCl	Periactin*	4 mg, 3-4 times/d	0.25 mg/kg, in 3-4 divided doses/d
SECOND-GENERATION (NONSEDATING OR MILDLY SEDATING) ANTIHISTAMINES			
Cetirizine HCl	Zyrtec†	5-10 mg qd	Available in tablets and syrup. 2-5 years: 2.5 mg qd; Max: 5 mg qd or 2.5 mg q 12 h; ≥6 years: 5-10 mg qd
Desloratadine	Clarinex†	5 mg qd	≥12 years: 5 mg qd
Loratadine	Claritin*†	10 mg qd	Available in tablet, syrup and reditab. ≥6 years: 10 mg qd; 2-5 years (syrup): 5 mg qd
Fexofenadine	Allegra†	60 mg bid or 180 mg once daily	≥12 years: 60 mg bid or 180 mg qd; twice daily or 180 mg once daily; 6-11 years: 30 mg bid
NASAL SPRAY ANTIHISTAMINES			
Azelastine HCl	Astelin Nasal Spray†	2 sprays per nostril bid years: 1 spray per nostril bid	≥12 years: 2 sprays per nostril bid; 5-11

* Over-the-counter preparation.
† Prescription only.

maceutical companies to combine them with oral decongestants.

The anticholinergic side effects of the first-generation antihistamines should be kept in mind also, particularly in treating older adults. The anticholinergic side effects include:

- Dry mouth
- Impotence
- Urinary hesitancy (especially in the elderly)
- Altered mental status.

Lack of the sedative side effect that occurs with the first-generation antihistamines is the main reason for the popularity of the second-generation antihistamines. Cetirizine is a derivative of hydroxyzine (a first-generation antihistamine). Cetirizine is considered mildly sedating.

The second-generation antihistamines classified as nonsedating are:

- Desloratadine
- Fexofenadine
- Loratadine.

The term "nonsedating" refers to the finding in controlled studies that subjects complained of no more sedation after treatment with the recommended dose of active drug than after placebo. However, some patients may still report a sedative effect with these agents.

■ Duration of Action

Both the first- and second-generation antihistamines demonstrate differences in duration of action. Among the first-generation agents, differences include:

- Brompheniramine—3 to 9 hours
- Chlorpheniramine—24 hours
- Diphenhydramine—3 to 9 hours
- Hydroxyzine—36 hours.

Differences of duration of action between the second-generation agents are:

- Fexofenadine—12 hours and 24 hours (the 24-hour fexofenadine is a new preparation that is long acting and is administered once a day)
- Loratadine, desloratadine, and cetirizine—24 hours.

■ Potency

Many of these data were obtained using an experimental model of cutaneous wheal suppression by the oral administration of these agents, which revealed apparent differences in their relative potency. Following is their ranking from most to least potent:

- Cetirizine
- Fexofenadine
- Desloratadine
- Loratadine
- Chlorpheniramine
- Placebo.

6

■ Adverse Events

Terfenadine (Seldane) and astemizole (Hismanal) are two antihistamines that have been withdrawn from the US market because of an association with cardiac arrhythmias (with rare fatalities), including >25 cases of torsades de pointes in the Food and Drug Administration (FDA) database. Terfenadine and astemizole may also affect the QT interval and cause prolongation in settings such as:

- Congenital QT prolongation
- Concomitant use of other antiarrhythmics:
  - Class IA (quinidine, procainamide, disopyramide)
  - Class III (amiodarone, sotalol)
- Electrolyte abnormalities
  - Hypomagnesemia
  - Hypokalemia.

Terfenadine was withdrawn from the market in 1998 after fexofenadine was introduced. Fexofenadine, also known as terfenadine carboxylate, received FDA-approval in 1996 because it lacked the adverse cardiovascular side effect of its parent drug. No QT prolongation has been seen even at high doses of fexofenadine. Fexofenadine has been shown to be effective in reducing symptoms of allergic rhinitis.

Astemizole was withdrawn from the market in 2000 because of its adverse cardiovascular side effects. An active metabolite of astemizole is currently under investigation (norastemizole).

■ Safety Issues

Second-generation antihistamines were developed because of the sedative properties of first-generation antihistamines. These new drugs are lyophobic and do not cross the blood-brain barrier, thereby avoiding the central nervous system effects seen with the first-generation antihistamines. Several states have ordinances that prohibit driving motor vehicles under the influence of sedating substances, including sedating antihistamines, and some antihistamines have warning labels to avoid machine operation as well as automobile driving with drug use. Current FDA guidelines allow only the use of fexofenadine and loratadine. Peer-reviewed guidelines on the diagnosis and management of allergic rhinitis by the American College of Allergy, Asthma, and Immunology (1998) recommend the use of second-generation antihistamines as first-line therapy for allergic rhinitis because of the improved safety profile and because there is some evidence that a few of the new H_1-antagonists may have antiasthma benefits.

Early reports in the 1970s suggested that antihistamines may be relatively contraindicated in patients with coexistent allergic rhinitis and bronchial asthma. This was based on the thought that excessive drying of the respiratory tract may exacerbate bronchospasm. However, subsequent experience in the last 10 to 15 years suggests that antihistamines are quite effective and safe for the symptomatic treatment of allergic rhinitis, even in patients with bronchial asthma. A position statement in 1988 by the American Academy of Allergy, Asthma, and Immunology (AAAAI) concludes that H_1-antagonist should be withheld from patients requiring antihistamines for concomitant diseases such as asthma, allergic rhinitis, allergic dermatoses, or urticaria. Loratadine, desloratadine, and cetirizine have been studied in patients with asthma and allergic rhinitis and both conditions have shown some benefit. Some factors to be considered among the second-generation antihistamines are listed in **Table 6.4**. In November 2002, the AAAAI issued a new position statement changing its stance to "antihistamines are not contraindicated in patients with asthma."

TABLE 6.4 — Factors to Be Considered Among the Second-Generation Antihistamines

	Sedation	Cardiac Effects
Azelastine	11.5%	No
Cetirizine 10 mg	13.7%	No
Desloratadine	No	No
Fexofenadine	No	No
Loratadine	No	No

■ Desloratadine

Desloratadine (Clarinex) is another second-generation selective oral antihistamine, released in 2002. It is the principal active metabolite of loratadine and has an elimination half-life of 27 hours, allowing for once-a-day dosing. Desloratadine is metabolized to 3-hydroxydesloratadine, and is absorbed well with or without food. It has approval for treatment of seasonal allergic rhinitis (SAR), perennial allergic rhinitis, and chronic idiopathic urticaria for patients ≥12 years of age. Clinical trials demonstrated efficacy and minimal side effects compared with placebo. There were no significant reports of sedation, cardiac effects, or negligible drug interactions.

This drug may also have some clinical advantages of decongestant activity as seen in three multicenter, double-blind, placebo-controlled trials and anti-inflammatory benefit seen with in vitro studies. There are no comparison studies with oral decongestants or inhaled steroids. Desloratadine has also been studied in patients with SAR and concomitant asthma, and two multicenter, double-blind, placebo-controlled studies have shown its benefit in decreasing total asthma symptoms and the use of β_2-agonists in patients with mild-to-moderate asthma who were previously using only albuterol for asthma medication. There was no improvement in the FEV_1.

■ Comparative Trials of Oral Antihistamines

Antihistamines relieve symptoms of allergic rhinitis. The majority of studies comparing first- and second-generation drugs show equal efficacy. Interestingly, there are two studies in which brompheniramine, a first-generation antihistamine, has provided better relief of symptoms when compared with loratadine and terfenadine. Brompheniramine did have more sedative side effects than the second-generation drugs. There is one published study (Van Cauwengerge and associates) comparing fexofenadine with loratadine. Six hundred eighty-eight patients with SAR were randomized in a multinational, double-blind, placebo-controlled, parallel-group study to evaluate efficacy, safety, and impact on quality of life. The dose of loratadine was 10 mg/d and fexofenadine was 120 mg/d. Fexofenadine was found to be significantly more effective than loratadine in decreasing nasal congestion and eye symptoms as well as in improving quality of life. However, there are two additional published double-blind, placebo-controlled trials comparing fexofenadine with loratadine that indicate loratadine provides greater relief of rhinitis symptoms than fexofenadine; these are in abstract form. Comparison between fexofenadine and cetirizine in the study by Howarth and associates showed no differences in efficacy of rhinitis symptoms, but cetirizine had a higher incidence of drowsiness and fatigue.

Several authors have assessed antihistamines on suppression of histamine-induced wheal and flare in the skin. Simons and colleagues found cetirizine 10 mg to be the most effective, followed by terfenadine 120 mg, terfenadine 60 mg, loratadine 10 mg, astemizole 10 mg, chlorpheniramine 4 mg, and placebo. Persi and associates compared cetirizine and loratadine with increasing grass-pollen nasal challenge and skin test response with grass allergen and histamine. Twenty-three patients completed the study. There was no significant difference seen between the two drugs with the nasal challenge, but cetirizine was more effective in suppressing histamine skin test response. Day and colleagues evaluated second-generation antihistamines in an environmental exposure unit with controlled ragweed-pollen exposure. Patients were given medications and their symptoms of rhinitis after ragweed exposure while in the unit were evaluated. Cetirizine was compared with loratadine in one study, and in another trial, cetirizine was compared with terfenadine, astemizole, loratadine, and placebo. Cetirizine was more effective than loratadine in reducing rhinitis symptoms in the first study. The second study demonstrated a higher efficacy ranking for cetirizine and terfenadine, followed by loratadine, astemizole, and placebo; however, these differences were not statistically significant ($P = 0.119$). Definitive relief and onset time for definitive relief did reveal significance between the drugs with the same ranking order. Desloratadine is the metabolite of loratadine. Anti-inflammatory action and intrinsic decongestant effects may be distinguishing properties of this antihistamine. Norastemizole is the metabolite of astemizole, and preliminary studies show no significant cardiotoxic effects.

In summary, trials have revealed little differences in relief of allergic rhinitis symptoms between the older and newer antihistamines, as well as little differences in efficacy between the second-generation antihistamines. Cetirizine has been shown to be more effective in suppressing histamine wheal and flare reaction in the skin. It also has a higher potential for sedation. Choosing an antihistamine will then depend upon cost and formulary restrictions, possible sedative effects, and patient preference.

Intranasal Antihistamines

Recently released for use in the United States as a nasal spray, the antihistamine azelastine (Astelin) provides a new medical option in the treatment of allergic rhinitis. It is formulated as a 0.1% liquid spray that allows rapid onset of action approximately 15 to 30 minutes after administration. Azelastine has shown relief of early-phase allergic symptoms such as sneezing, rhinorrhea, and itching as well as benefit in reducing nasal congestion, a late-phase symptom. Adverse side effects of bitter taste (metallic) and somnolence are reported in a small percentage of patients (19.7% and 11.5%, respectively).

There is a US study (Banov and Lieberman, 2001) demonstrating benefit in reduction of symptoms of vasomotor rhinitis with the use of topical azelastine. This trial has led to a new indication for azelastine. The drug is approved for the treatment of SAR and nonallergic vasomotor rhinitis. Anti-inflammatory effects seen with azelastine include decreased neutrophils and eosinophils in both the immediate and late allergic phases as well as lowered levels of leukotrienes and kinins after nasal allergen challenge. These actions may explain azelastine's beneficial effects on nasal congestion and vasomotor rhinitis. There are two reported studies comparing azelastine with intranasal steroids. One study (Pelucchi A and associates, 1995) demonstrated equal efficacy between azelastine and beclomethasone for reduction of symptoms of allergic rhinitis. The second study (Stern MA and associates, 1998) found budesonide to be superior to azelastine in decreasing perennial allergic rhinitis symptoms.

■ Comparison of Intranasal Antihistamines and Oral Antihistamines

There have been two studies comparing oral antihistamines and azelastine. Berger and colleagues demonstrated significant improvement with azelastine with the total nasal-symptom complex in SAR patients who continued to be symptomatic (<25% improvement) after 1 week of treatment with loratadine 10 mg. Patients were randomized to azelastine nasal spray 2 sprays bid; azelastine with loratadine 10 mg; desloratadine 5 mg; or placebo. Patients improved after 2 weeks of therapy with azelastine alone, azelastine with loratadine, and desloratadine compared with placebo. No additional benefit was seen when azelastine was used in combination with loratadine. Desloratadine only improved sneezing symptoms significantly when compared with placebo.

A follow-up study was performed demonstrating efficacy of azelastine as monotherapy in patients who remained symptomatic after treatment with fexofenadine. This study was also a multicenter, randomized, double-blind placebo-controlled 2-week study in patients with SAR. Patients received fexofenadine 60 mg bid during a 1-week, open-label, lead-in period.

Patients who improved <25% with fexofenadine were then randomized to azelastine nasal spray 2 sprays bid; azelastine nasal spray 2 sprays bid and fexofenadine 60 mg bid; or placebo for 2 weeks. After 2 weeks, azelastine spray and azelastine spray with fexofenadine significantly improved total nasal-symptom score compared with placebo. The study also found azelastine spray monotherapy to be as effective as the dual therapy of azelastine and fexofenadine.

■ Comparison of Intranasal Antihistamines and Intranasal Corticosteroids

Several articles have compared intranasal steroid sprays with the available topical antihistamine nasal sprays. A recent meta-analysis of the randomized controlled trials focused on the use of intranasal corticosteroid sprays vs intranasal antihistamines in the treatment of allergic rhinitis. The meta-analysis reviewed nine studies and found that the intranasal steroid sprays relieved nasal symptoms of sneezing, rhinorrhea, itching, and nasal congestion to a significant degree compared with the topical antihistamines. The topical antihistamines that were studied were azelastine and levocabastine (presently not available in the United States). The study concluded that intranasal steroid sprays were more effective in the treatment of allergic rhinitis with regard to nasal symptoms compared with the intranasal antihistamines.

Azelastine nasal spray should be considered for individuals who have adverse reactions to oral antihistamines as well as those who do not tolerate intranasal corticosteroid sprays.

In summary, azelastine nasal spray is a unique treatment modality in the armamentarium of drugs used to treat both allergic and nonallergic rhinitis. It is quick in onset, long-lasting in duration, and can be administered regularly or as needed. It is the only intranasal antihistamine spray available on the market and can decrease nasal congestion as well as provide the usual antihistamine benefits.

Decongestants

Nasal congestion is one of the most common complaints of patients with chronic rhinitis and because antihistamines do not adequately relieve nasal congestion, additional intervention is often needed. If obstruction is intermittent and cannot be attributed to the shape of nasal bone and cartilage, thickness of the soft tissues of the nose is probably caused by edema of the mucosa and engorgement of the venous sinusoids. Decongestant nasal sprays reduce the amount of blood in the venous sinusoids, thereby reducing the volume of space occupied by the turbinates.

■ Nasal Sprays

Available nasal sprays include the α-agonists (**Table 6.5**):

- Phenylephrine
- Oxymetazoline
- Xylometazoline
- Naphazoline.

When used for more than 5 to 7 consecutive days, however, these potent vasoconstrictors are associated with the development of rebound congestion on withdrawal. Prolonged use leads to rhinitis medicamentosa. Thus the topical decongestants may be used for acute viral rhinitis but not for allergic rhinitis, which has an expected duration of weeks or months.

■ Oral Decongestants

The oral decongestant pseudoephedrine is commonly combined with antihistamines to improve relief from nasal congestion. Principal side effects are:

- Nervousness

TABLE 6.5 — Over-the-Counter Decongestants

Generic Name	Trade Name	Delivery Device	Dosage (Adults)
INHALED SYMPATHOMIMETICS — *Short-Acting*			
Ephedrine hydrochloride	Efedron Gel	Nasal jelly	Small amount/nostril q 4 h
Naphazoline hydrochloride	Privine	Drops	1-2 drops/nostril q 3-4 h prn
		Sprays	1-2 sprays/nostril q 3-4 h prn
Phenylephrine hydrochloride	Duration, Neo-Synephrine, Nostril, Vicks-Sinex, others	Spray or drops	1-2 sprays/nostril q 4 h prn
Tetrahydrozoline hydrochloride	Tyzine	Solution	2-4 drops/nostril q 4-6 h prn
INHALED SYMPATHOMIMETICS — *Long-Acting*			
Oxymetazoline hydrochloride	Afrin, Decongest, Dristan Long-Lasting, Neo-Synephrine 12-Hour, Neo-Synephrine Maximum Strength, Nostrilla, others	Spray or drops	2-4 sprays/nostril bid
Xylometazoline hydrochloride	Otrivin	Drops	2-3 drops/nostril q 8-10 h
		Spray	1-2 sprays/nostril q 8-10 h
	Sinex Long-Acting	Spray	1-2 sprays/nostril q 8-10 h

ORAL SYMPATHOMIMETICS			
Pseudoephedrine hydrochloride	Novafed	Capsule	120 mg (1 capsule) po q 12 h
	Pseudogest	Syrup	60 mg (2 tsp) po q 4 h
		Tablet	60 mg po q 4 h
	Sudafed	Tablet	60 mg po q 4 h
	Sudafed 12-Hour	Tablet	120 mg po q 12 h
HYBRID INTRANASAL SPRAYS			
Phenylephrine HCL/naphazoline HCL/pyrilamine maleate	4-Way Fast-Acting	Nasal spray metered pump	1-2 sprays/nostril q 3-4 h
Phenylephrine HCL/ pheniramine maleate	Dristan Nasal	Nasal spray	1-2 sprays/nostril q 3-4 h
Phenylephine HCL/ pyrilamine maleate	MYCl Spray	Nasal spray	1-2 sprays/nostril q 3-4 h

6

- Insomnia
- Irritability
- Headache
- Palpitations
- Tachycardia.

Oral decongestants may interfere with urinary flow in males and are contraindicated in patients with:

- Hypertension
- Severe coronary artery disease
- Monoamine oxidase inhibitor (MAOI) therapy.

Prolonged use of oral decongestants on a daily basis may lead to withdrawal symptoms of headache and fatigue when the drug is stopped.

■ Phenylpropanolamine

The FDA has recalled the over-the-counter use of phenylpropanolamine in cold and cough remedies and in appetite suppressants. Kernan and associates identified the drug as a risk factor for hemorrhagic stroke in women in a case-control study of 702 men and women ages 18 to 49 years old. Currently, there are no case-control studies on the safety of ephedrine, pseudoephrine, and phenylephrine. It is advised that the other available decongestant preparations be used with caution.

Intranasal Corticosteroids

Corticosteroids require hours to take effect due to the many intracellular and intranuclear events necessary to produce posttranscriptional proteins. In turn, these proteins inhibit multiple steps in the inflammatory process. As summarized by Meltzer, they:

- Cause vasoconstriction
- Decrease glandular response to cholinergic stimulation

- Interfere with arachidonic acid metabolism
- Reduce mediator release
- Decrease production of cytokines from T_{H2} lymphocytes
- Inhibit influx of eosinophils to the nasal epithelium.

Topical nasal steroid sprays, which are the most potent medications available for the treatment of allergic rhinitis, include (**Table 6.6**):

- Beclomethasone
- Budesonide
- Dexamethasone
- Flunisolide
- Fluticasone
- Mometasone
- Triamcinolone acetonide.

6

Budesonide and fluticasone are the most topically potent, according to a vasoconstrictor index of potency (**Table 6.7**). While mometasone was not studied in this manner, one can speculate it has similar potency to budesomide and fluticasone.

Nasal steroid sprays effectively reduce nasal mucosal congestion, sneezing, and rhinorrhea, but they must be combined with antihistamine to effectively control eye symptoms. Both aqueous pump spray and pressurized aerosol forms are available.

■ Onset and Duration of Action

Older intranasal corticosteroid medications, such as beclomethasone, flunisolide, and triamcinolone, have not been well studied to determine their onset of action. Previous information suggests onset within 3 days. Fluticasone and mometasone have shown some relief of nasal symptoms by 7 to 12 hours. Differences between the intranasal corticosteroids are also seen with recommendations for dosing. The more potent

TABLE 6.6 — Steroid Nasal Inhalers/Sprays

Generic Name	Trade Name	Delivery Device	Dosage (Adults)
Beclomethasone dipropionate	Beconase AQ	Pump spray	1-2 sprays/nostril bid (42 µg/spray)
	Vancenase AQ DS	Pump spray	1-2 sprays/nostril qd (84 µg/spray)
	Vancenase Pockethaler	Aerosol inhaler	1 spray/nostril bid-qid (42 µg/spray)
Budesonide	Rhinocort AQ	Pump spray	1 spray/nostril qd (32 µg/spray)
Flunisolide	Nasalide	Pump spray	2 sprays/nostril bid (25 µg/spray)
	Nasarel	Pump spray	2 sprays/nostril bid (25 µg/spray)
Fluticasone propionate	Flonase	Pump spray	2 sprays/nostril qd (50 µg/spray)
Mometasone furoate monohydrate	Nasonex	Pump spray	2 sprays/nostril qd (50 µg/spray)
Triamcinolone acetonide	Nasacort AQ	Pump spray	2 sprays/nostril qd (55 µg/spray)

TABLE 6.7 — Relative Topical Vasoconstrictor Potency	
Drug	**Activity**
Hydrocortisone	1
Triamcinolone	1,000
Flunisolide	3,000
Beclomethasone	5,000
Budesonide	10,000
Fluticasone	10,000

Modified from: Meltzer EO. *J Allergy Clin Immunol.* 1995; 95:1097-1110; and Siegel SC. *J Allergy Clin Immunol.* 1988; 81:984-991.

6

corticosteroids are administered once a day, whereas the others are given bid or qid.

Dykewicz and associates performed a 4-week, multicenter, randomized, double-blind, placebo-controlled study with fluticasone nasal spray 200 μg 2 sprays in each nostril used as needed once a day in 241 SAR patients. Patients used fluticasone a mean of 61.8% days and had a significantly greater reduction from total nasal-symptom score baseline compared with vehicle placebo. Patients randomized to placebo spray used the spray a mean of 70.1% days. Adverse side effects were comparable between the two groups and included headache, sore throat, diarrhea, and odontalgia. Epistaxis occurred in 2% of patients treated with fluticasone compared with 0% of patients using placebo. The authors suggest that the safety data for prn use of fluticasone may reveal a lower incidence of adverse side effects compared with regular and daily use of the spray.

■ Potency

Potency of corticosteroids can be measured by binding affinity of the steroid compound to the glucocorticoid receptor as well as by relative topical vasoconstrictor index. Budesonide, fluticasone, and mometasone appear to have the most potent activity (**Table 6.8**).

■ Adverse Effects

Local adverse side effects have been reported with intranasal corticosteroids. These are most commonly nasal irritation or dryness and epistaxis. The nasal bleeding may be minimized by directing the spray away from the septum and by using lower-velocity sprays. Excipients, or inactive components, in the intranasal steroid sprays may also cause local side effects. Septal perforation has also been reported as a rare side effect of nasal steroid sprays and may be associated with use of topical decongestant sprays as well as improper application of the medication to the septum.

Systemic side effects result from the swallowed portion of intranasal sprays as well as the amount of drug absorbed through the nasal mucosa. Given the sprays' low systemic absorption and first-pass metabolism through the liver, there is minimal evidence for systemic effects within the dosage ranges recommended by the manufacturers. The older dexamethasone spray does have significant suppressive effect on adrenal function.

Use of intranasal steroid sprays in children has been approved by the FDA. There is a warning in the prescription information of possible adverse growth effects when the drug is administered to children long term. Short-term studies with mometasone, fluticasone, and budesonide have not shown growth suppression. Long-term use of nasal steroids has shown no significant deleterious effects on nasal mucosa (1-year-duration studies for fluticasone and mometasone, a 5.5-

TABLE 6.8 — Clinically Distinguishing Factors of Newer Intranasal Steroids

Medication	Onset of Action	Systemic Availability (%)	Relative GR-Binding Affinity*
Beclomethasone dipropionate	Within 3 days	17	NA
Budesonide	In 24 hours, generally within a few days	11	258
Flunisolide	4 to 7 days	20-50	NA
Fluticasone propionate	12 hours to several days	<2	813
Mometasone furoate	Median 35.9 hours, begins within 12 hours	<0.1	1235
Triamcinolone acetonide	May occur as early as 24 hours; 7 days (maximum benefit)	22	164

Abbreviation: NA, not available.

* Relative binding affinity was expressed as reciprocal of relative amount of test ligand needed to replace 50% of bound tritiated dexamethasone, which represented positive control with binding affinity of 100.

Adapted from: Lumry WR. *J Allergy Cin Immunol.* 1999;104:150-158.

year study for budesonide). There is some evidence to suggest that the regular use of these medications may reverse some allergen-induced inflammatory pathologic changes as well. Nasal candidiasis has not been an issue with the nasal steroids. Development of cataracts and glaucoma with long-term use of intranasal steroid sprays has not been confirmed in a prospective manner at this time.

■ Comparative Trials of Intranasal Corticosteroid Sprays

All symptoms of allergic rhinitis, which include sneezing, itching, rhinorrhea, and nasal congestion, are reduced with the use of intranasal steroid sprays. Comparative trials have been performed between fluticasone vs beclomethasone, fluticasone vs budesonide, fluticasone vs triamcinolone. Mometasone has been compared with fluticasone and with beclomethasone. Surprisingly, little difference has been shown in efficacy for control of rhinitis symptoms between the older steroid agents (beclomethasone, triamcinolone) and the newer agents (budesonide, fluticasone, and mometasone). Studies comparing budesonide, fluticasone, and mometasone also indicate comparable efficacy.

Mandl's article compares mometasone and fluticasone in a multinational, randomized, double-blind, double-dummy, parallel-group study. The two drugs were found to be equal in efficacy in 459 patients with perennial rhinitis. Stern and colleagues compared aqueous budesonide at 128 μg (4 puffs/d) and 256 μg (8 puffs/d) with fluticasone 200 μg (4 puffs/d) in 635 adult patients. The study found budesonide at 256 μg/d to be more effective than fluticasone 200 μg/d and budesonide 128 μg/d, especially on high pollen–count days. These results were confirmed by Day and associates again when comparing aqueous budesonide at the dose of 256 μg to fluticasone 200 μg. Another study by Andersson and colleagues compared budesonide dry-powder spray at doses of 200 μg/d. This study did not find any significant differences in efficacy between the two doses of budesonide and fluticasone.

While older steroid agents have slower onset of action and higher systemic availability, they have proven to be clinically similar to the newer agents in controlling symptoms of rhinitis. Budesonide, fluticasone, and mometasone have lower systemic bioavailability (11%, <2%, <1%, respectively) and have demonstrated quick onset of action in ≥24 hours. Another differentiating aspect between older and newer steroid sprays is dosing frequency. Juniper and colleagues studied prn use of the older class of steroid, beclomethasone, in 60 adult patients with ragweed rhinitis. The study revealed that regular use of beclomethasone controlled symptoms better than prn use but that this difference did not approach statistical significance. Jen and associates found fluticasone to be effective when used on a prn basis in the management of SAR. Eosinophils in nasal lavage were also found to be significantly lower in the active group treated with medication compared with placebo. Once-a-day dosing or prn dosing obviously improves patient compliance and use.

A meta-analysis was published in the *Journal of Laryngology and Otology* in November 2003 in which Waddell and associates compared available intranasal steroid sprays in the United Kingdom. The authors reviewed eight articles to determine comparative efficacy of available intranasal steroids. They state: "There is no clear evidence to support the suggestion that one particular steroid spray is more effective than another in the treatment of seasonal allergic rhinitis or perennial allergic rhinitis." The analysis compared local and systematic adverse side effects for all available intranasal steroids. Epistaxis was the most common side effect noted with all of the sprays with a reported incidence of 17% to 23%. Comparing systemic adverse effects, the authors cite one article (Wilson A and associates, 1998) that reported fluticasone to cause a significant reduction in endogenous cortisol secretion, while triamcinolone, beclomethasone, budesonide, and mometasone did not. The article also reported that there is little evidence that intranasal steroids affect skeletal growth.

■ Comparative Trials of Intranasal Steroid Sprays and Oral Antihistamines

Recommendations from the ARIA guidelines and from the Joint Task Force on Practice Parameters for Allergic Rhinitis state that oral antihistamines and intranasal corticosteroid sprays are first-line therapy for the treatment of allergic rhinitis. A meta-analysis was published by Weiner and colleagues in the *British Medical Journal* 1998. The authors' objectives were to determine if intranasal steroid sprays were more effective than oral antihistamines in the treatment of allergic rhinitis. The end point that was evaluated was comparison of relief of nasal symptoms. The authors identified 16 randomized controlled trials and concluded that the intranasal steroid sprays provided more relief than oral antihistamines with regard to sneezing, nasal itching, nasal discharge, postnasal drip, and nasal congestion. They found that there was no significant difference in outcome measures of eye symptoms. The authors concluded that results of their meta-analysis support the use of intranasal corticosteroid sprays over the use of oral antihistamines while also considering safety and cost effectiveness factors. This study recommended intranasal steroid sprays as a first-line treatment for allergic rhinitis.

Another review of randomized controlled trials between intranasal steroids and antihistamines was published in *American Journal of Respiratory Medi-*

cine in 2003 by Neilson and Dahl. These authors also found that the literature supports use of intranasal steroids compared with antihistamines with regard to efficacy and that there were no significant differences in safety data between the two classes of medication.

■ Choosing an Intranasal Steroid Spray

An ideal nasal steroid spray would demonstrate quick onset of action, high potency, low systemic side effects, infrequent dosing, and low incidence of local side effects. All preparations of nasal steroid sprays are effective. While older sprays are initially administered more frequently than once a day, dosing may be decreased after symptoms are under control. Other factors that may influence choice of nasal steroid agent include wet (liquid) vs dry (powder) spray (if available), volume of spray, and odor or taste of the preparation. Nonbiased comparative trials of all intranasal steroids assessing patient preferences and sensory properties of the steroid preparations would be helpful for physicians to select a particular nasal steroid spray. Cost of nasal steroid spray is also a factor, and some insurance plans preselect medications that may be prescribed; otherwise, patients may incur additional costs. Compared with the nonsedating antihistamines, intranasal sprays tend to be slightly lower in cost.

■ Other Uses of Intranasal Steroid Sprays

Intranasal steroid sprays have been administered in nasal diseases other than rhinitis. Some studies have indicated benefit from steroid sprays when used as adjunctive therapy for acute and chronic sinusitis, as well as nasal polyposis. Although there is no FDA indication at this time for nasal steroids in these conditions, the known anti-inflammatory properties of corticosteroids provide rationale for their use.

Cromolyn Sodium

Cromolyn sodium is effective for symptomatic control of both SAR and perennial allergic rhinitis. In general, cromolyn sodium should be administered prophylactically before exposure; it can prevent both the acute and late-phase reactions to allergen. Although effective, it is less potent than nasal corticosteroids. The safety profile of cromolyn sodium is excellent. Delivered by metered inhaler, cromolyn sodium dosage is one spray/nostril qid before onset of nasal symptoms. The medication is now available over the counter. **Table 6.9** lists miscellaneous agents for rhinitis.

Anticholinergics

Anticholinergics are known to be drying agents. Ipratropium bromide (Atrovent) nasal spray is currently the only topical anticholinergic agent available. Rhinorrhea is predominantly cholinergically mediated, and ipratropium blocks the hypersecretory effects of the cholinergic neurotransmitter acetylcholine by competing with it for binding sites on the cell.

Ipratropium nasal spray is equally effective against the rhinorrhea associated with allergic and nonallergic rhinitis and the common cold. When compared with nasal saline, which can itself be beneficial in the treatment of rhinitis, ipratropium therapy resulted in a 30% reduction in rhinorrhea. Less-significant reductions were seen in postnasal drip, congestion, and sneezing. Preliminary data suggest that, when combined with antihistamines or corticosteroids, ipratropium produces additional control of rhinorrhea without added side effects.

In common-cold studies, onset of action was within 1 hour. No rebound in rhinorrhea was seen following discontinuation of ipratropium. The nasal spray maintains its effectiveness in long-term use and may

TABLE 6.9 — Miscellaneous Agents for Rhinitis

Generic Name	Trade Name	Delivery Device	Dosage (Adults)
Cromolyn solution	Nasalcrom*	Solution (metered inhaler)	1 spray/nostril tid-qid up to 6/d
Ipratropium bromide	Atrovent Nasal Spray	Metered-dose pump spray (0.03%)	2 sprays/nostril bid-tid (21 µg/spray)
		Metered-dose pump spray (0.06%)	2 sprays/nostril tid-qid (42 µg/spray)
Montelukast	Singulair	Tablet	1 10-mg tablet/d (for pediatric patients 6-14 years of age: 1 5-mg chewable tablet daily; 2-5 years of age: 1 4-mg chewable tablet or 1 packet of 4-mg oral granules daily)

* Over-the-counter preparation.

reduce the need for concomitant rhinitis medications. Ipratropium does not cause systemic anticholinergic side effects when administered topically. Dryness of the nose and mouth may occur but can be controlled with a reduction in dosage.

Ipratropium nasal spray comes in two strengths:

- 0.03% for chronic therapy in allergic and nonallergic rhinitis, dosage, 2 sprays (42 µg/nostril) bid-tid
- 0.06% for acute therapy in the common cold, dosage, 2 sprays (84 µg/nostril) tid-qid.

It is the only approved prescription nasal spray for the control of rhinorrhea in colds. It has also been helpful in other refractory conditions, such as gustatory rhinitis.

Leukotriene Receptor Antagonist

■ Montelukast

Montelukast was approved by the FDA in 2003 for the treatment of SAR in pediatric patients >2 years of age (**Table 6.9**). It had previously been approved for the treatment of asthma. The drug is a leukotriene-receptor antagonist that inhibits cysteinyl leukotrienes from binding to respiratory tract receptors. Cysteinyl leukotrienes are proinflammatory mediators that are released from mast cells that induce symptoms of allergic rhinitis. Montelukast has a half-life of 4.9 hours and is metabolized in the liver by CYP3A4.

Several randomized, double-blind, placebo-controlled studies have found that montelukast decreased symptoms of SAR more than placebo. These trials enrolled >2500 patients. Three comparative studies of montelukast vs intranasal steroid sprays have found fluticasone propionate more effective in controlling SAR symptoms compared with montelukast. There were no significant adverse effects reported with montelukast.

Two studies reviewed the use of leukotriene receptors in the treatment of allergic rhinitis. A study by Nathan reviewed the pathophysiology of allergic rhinitis and employed a search for articles comparing leukotriene-receptor antagonists to other medications used in the treatment of allergic rhinitis. The second article, published in the *American Journal of Medicine*, reviewed 11 studies that compared leukotriene-receptor antagonists vs placebo or other treatments. Included are three studies that reviewed leukotriene-receptor antagonists with an antihistamine. The authors found that:

- Leukotriene-receptor antagonists were better than placebo
- Leukotrienes were as effective as antihistamines
- Nasal steroid sprays were the most effective in improving total nasal-symptom scores and quality of life.

Ocular Therapy

Ocular itching and watering nearly always accompany nasal symptoms in allergic rhinitis. Steroids are not suitable for topical ocular use because of the risk of ocular infection and cataracts. Thus oral antihistamines are the agents of choice for ocular itching.

The topical antihistamine pheniramine maleate in combination with the vasoconstrictor naphazoline is available for temporary relief of eye symptoms. Rebound congestion has also been noted in the eyes with the use of ocular decongestants. Given systemic absorption of the vasoconstrictor, however, the combination should be avoided in patients with severe cardiovascular disease.

The antihistamine levocabastine hydrochloride is available for topical use and has compared favorably with oral terfenadine in control of ocular itching. The effect of levocabastine is immediate in contrast to that of cromolyn sodium or lodoxamide, which may take several days to be effective. Transient stinging of the eyes is a problem as with many ocular medications. The preservative benzalkonium chloride can damage contact lenses.

Cromolyn sodium ophthalmic drops, administered four to six times a day, are effective in reducing ocular itching, inflammation, and discharge. Full effect of the drug may not be seen for a week or more. A recent addition to ocular therapy is ketotifen, known as a second-generation antihistamine with mast-cell stabilizing actions similar to those of cromolyn sodium, but it has been released only for use in vernal keratoconjunctivitis.

A nonsteroidal anti-inflammatory drug, ketorolac, has also been released for treatment of allergic conjunctivitis. At the recommended qid dosing, ocular irritation is common. Olopatadine is the first drug indicated for the prevention of itching due to allergic conjunctivitis (in adults and children >3 years old) that both inhibits mast-cell degranulation and is a selective histamine H_1-receptor antagonist. **Table 6.10** lists the available ocular agents.

Anti-IgE Monoclonal Antibody

An antihuman immunoglobulin E (IgE) monoclonal antibody (omalizumab [Xolair]) has been studied in atopic patients with asthma, as well as in patients with allergic rhinitis. The anti-IgE binds to circulating serum IgE, decreasing the level of IgE to bind to mast cell surface receptors. Preliminary results show decrease in nasal and ocular allergic symptoms compared with placebo. This product is administered monthly as an injection to reduce symptoms of IgE

TABLE 6.10 — Ophthalmic Agents	
Generic Name	**Trade Name**
Azelastine hydrochloride	Optivar
Cromolyn sodium	Opticrom
Ketorolac tromethamine	Acular
Ketotifen fumarate	Zaditor
Levocabastine	Livostin
Loteprednol	Alrex
Nedocromil sodium	Alocril
Olopatadine hydrochloride	Patanol
Pemirolast potassium	Alamast

overload in severe asthmatics. For a complete discussion, see Chapter 8, *Coexistence of Rhinitis and Asthma*.

Pregnancy and Asthma/ Allergy Medications

The FDA has published guidelines for prescribing asthma/allergy medications for pregnant patients. Drugs are classified into four groups, A through D, based on available data regarding relative risk. Most asthma and allergy medications are classified as B or C risks. Those classified as group D, which should not be prescribed during pregnancy, are:

- Tetracycline
- Iodide-containing expectorants.

A list of asthma/allergy medications and FDA risk-factor ratings are summarized in **Table 6.11**.

TABLE 6.11 — Risk to Fetus of Allergy and Asthma Medications During Pregnancy

	Risk Factor Category
Bronchodilator	
Terbutaline	B
Albuterol	C
Foradil	C
Metaproterenol	C
Salmeterol	C
Theophylline	C
Anti-inflammatory	
Cromolyn sodium	B
Montelukast	B
Nedocromil sodium	B
Zafirlukast	B
Beclomethasone dipropionate	C
Budesonide	B/C
Flunisolide	C
Mometasone	C
Fluticasone	C
Triamcinolone	C
Zileuton	C
Prednisone	(Not rated)
Antihistamine	
Cetirizine	B
Chlorpheniramine	B
Diphenhydramine	B
Loratadine	B
Triprolidine	B
Azelastine	C
Brompheniramine	C
Desloratadine	C
Fexofenadine	C

Key to Risk Factor Ratings

(According to Manufacturer's FDA-Approved Product Labeling)

A **Controlled studies show no risk**. Adequate, well-controlled studies in pregnant women have failed to demonstrate risk to the fetus.

B **No evidence of risk in humans**. Either animal findings show risk but human findings do not; or if no adequate human studies have been done, animal findings are negative.

Continued

C	**Risk cannot be ruled out**. Human studies are lacking, and animal studies are either positive for fetal risk or lacking as well. However, potential benefits may justify the potential risk.
D	**Positive evidence of risk**. Investigational or postmarketing data show risk to the fetus. Nevertheless, potential benefits may outweigh the potential risk.
X	**Contraindicated in pregnancy**. Studies in animals or humans, or investigational or postmarketing reports, have shown fetal risk that clearly outweighs any possible benefit to the patient.

Modified and reproduced from: National Heart, Lung, and Blood Institute. National Asthma Education and Prevention Program. Expert Panel Report 2. Guidelines for the diagnosis and management of asthma. Bethesda, Md: National Institutes of Health; 1997. Publication no. 97-4051.

Future Therapeutic Options

■ Antihistamines

Norastemizole is a new antihistamine that is being developed at this time. Norastemizole is the metabolite of astemizole, and preliminary studies show no significant cardiotoxic effects.

Topical mast-cell inhibitors are soon to be released. These include ketotifen and olopatidine nasal sprays. These medications are currently well recognized as ophthalmologic products that are safe and effective. They will be utilized as adjunctive management in patients with allergic nasal disorders.

■ Leukotriene-Receptor Antagonist

Another leukotriene inhibitor will be reintroduced to the market: zileuton. This product had limited success earlier due to compliance issues, however, the new formulation will enhance the compliance issues and may prove to assist with reduction of patient symptoms.

■ Anticytokine Therapy

Interleukin (IL)-4 and IL-5 have been identified as important cytokines in allergic inflammatory diseases. Agents that can modulate these cytokines are now being studied in the treatment of asthma and may have a role in the future therapy of allergic rhinitis.

7 Rhinitis: Immunotherapy

Immunotherapy is reserved for patients with allergic rhinitis and conjunctivitis whose symptoms cannot be adequately controlled with antihistamines and nasal steroid sprays. For those with isolated allergy to ragweed, immunotherapy is usually not needed since the season lasts only a few weeks each year. The extracts used in immunotherapy, which include pollen, house-dust mite, cat, and some molds, reduce symptoms and sensitivity to nasal or bronchial provocation.

Most allergic rhinitis patients are sensitive to multiple pollens. Thus someone with allergy to tree, grass, and weed pollens has symptoms for 6 to 9 months of the year, and in some parts of the country, grass season extends throughout the year. For patients who have been sensitized to house-dust mites as well as pollens, immunotherapy provides relief from nearly year-round symptoms while reducing medication requirements. Immunotherapy provides 80% of appropriately selected patients with 50% to 75% relief from symptoms of allergic rhinitis and conjunctivitis.

The beneficial response to immunotherapy is dose-related. Since doses near to maximum toleration are needed to produce benefit, local reactions at the site of injection are common and systemic reactions are always a possibility. Thus any facility giving allergy shots must be prepared to treat reactions, including anaphylaxis.

Part of the immunologic response to immunotherapy is the production of immunoglobulin G (IgG)–specific antibody to the allergen injected. According to one theory, the newly generated IgG does not fix to mast cells but can react with antigen diffusing into tissues. The IgG response develops slowly, reaching a maximum after several months of shots. Allergy shots may be given in the allergy specialist's or primary care physician's office, but should not be given at home, since the person giving the shot must be fully prepared to treat anaphylaxis. Systemic allergic reactions can occur at any point in the initiation, buildup, or maintenance of the therapeutic course. Strict attention must be paid to appropriate extracts as well as the correct dose for each patient. The date of each shot and notation of any local or systemic symptoms must be recorded.

The interval between shots is also important. For example, because blocking antibody, which is thought to play an important role in the tolerance for the shots, has a half-life of less than a month, a shot interval of 2 months requires a major reduction in the next allergy shot. The protective nature of allergy shots has been emphasized recently, with the proposal to refer to allergy extracts as allergy vaccines. Currently, as a result of standardization, the preparation of these extracts or vaccines is more complicated than ever. For many years, extracts have been used in weight-by-volume concentrations. The realization that this did not correlate reliably with the allergic potency resulted in a number of efforts to standardize extracts. Ragweed extract may still be sold in weight-by-volume vials. Dust mite allergen extract is sold in allergy units/cc (AU/cc). Cat allergen extract is sold in biologic allergy units/cc (BAU/cc), as are grass pollens. A 10,000-BAU/cc vial is 10 times more concentrated than a tree pollen of 1/10,000. A complex immunotherapy program may contain extracts using a variety of concentration units.

Allergy shots are given in gradually increasing doses as tolerance increases. Early in the program, dilute extracts are used. The maintenance concentration may be 100× to 1000× initially, but by the time the maintenance dose is reached, the patient tolerates environmental exposure to the allergen as well. Maintenance shots are continued at intervals of every 2 to 4 weeks throughout the year. Allergic patients are continued on the shots until they have been essentially free of rhinitis and conjunctivitis symptoms for two seasons. The goal of both pharmacologic therapy and immunotherapy is to allow patients with allergic rhinitis to enjoy normal activities indoors and outdoors with a minimum of symptoms.

8 Coexistence of Rhinitis and Asthma

There is an emerging view that allergic rhinitis and asthma are similar pathophysiologic processes that occur in the upper and lower airways and form a continuum rather than being distinct entities (**Table 8.1**). Several lines of evidence support this notion:

- Epidemiologic data show a frequent coexistence of both rhinitis and asthma.
- Immunologic processes that are present are similar and active in both entities (both cells and mediators).
- Local provocation studies (ie, nasal allergen challenge or bronchial segmental allergen challenge) trigger de novo symptoms and inflammation in the unchallenged area.
- Clinical studies indicate that therapy for rhinitis improves asthma control when the two diseases are coexistent.
- Allergy is a systemic disease that involves precursor cells from the bone marrow and several target organs, including upper airway nasal passages as well as the lower airway (**Figure 8.1**).

A large body of both experimental and clinical studies over the past decade has contributed to a new paradigm that has been variously referred to as united airways disease, single airway disease, allergic rhinobronchitis, or composite airway disease (**Figure 8.2**). There are several therapeutic implications to this reasoning, including:

- Optimal treatment of rhinitis is important in and of itself.

TABLE 8.1 — Theories Regarding the Link Between Rhinitis and Asthma

Possibilities

- Allergic responses to allergen induce a systemic immune response involving bone marrow progenitors that populate the nose and bronchi with eosinophils, basophils, granulocytes, and monocytes
- Absorption of mediators and immune reactants derived from the nose and sinuses that cause up-regulation of pulmonary immune responses and clinical asthma
- Increased oral breathing in the presence of nasal/sinus disease
- Infection of the nasopharynx with spread to bronchi and a pulmonary immune response (rhinovirus)
- Nasal-bronchial reflex?
- Postnasal drainage affecting patients with asthma

Disproved

- Aspiration of nasal secretions with an intact cough reflex

Greenberger PA. *Allergy Asthma Proc*. 2004;25:89-93.

- Asthma is a serious disease that has significant morbidity and treatment of coexistent rhinitis helps asthma outcomes.

A variety of both cross-sectional as well as longitudinal studies have demonstrated a coexistence between allergic rhinitis and asthma. Cross-sectional studies indicate that 40% to 50% of patients with allergic rhinitis have coexistent asthma compared with a background prevalence of asthma in 5% to 10% of the general population based on data from several studies around the world. On the other hand, the prevalence of allergic rhinitis among patients with diagnosed asthma is as high as 80% to 90%. Longitudinal studies have indicated that the presence of allergic rhinitis alone involves a 3-fold risk for the development of

FIGURE 8.1 — Summary of the Hypotheses Explaining the Links Between Rhinitis and Asthma

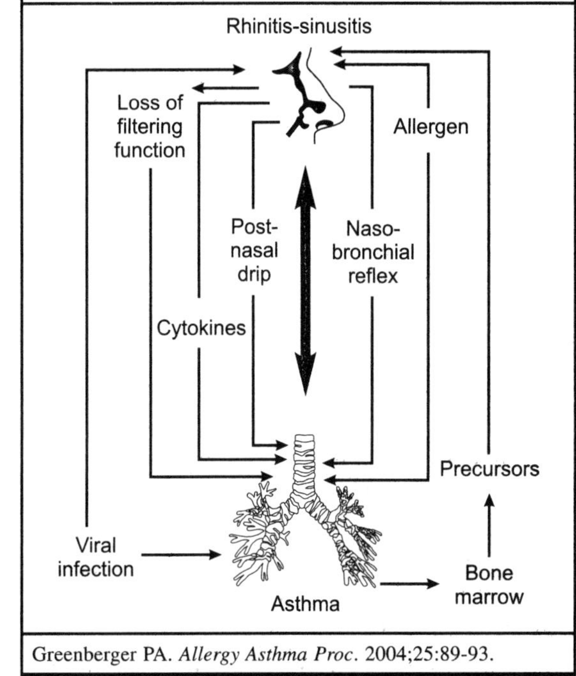

Greenberger PA. *Allergy Asthma Proc.* 2004;25:89-93.

asthma later in life. Studies indicate that rhinitis usually precedes asthma as a risk factor for developing asthma independent of atopic status. Epidemiologic studies also suggest a common occurrence of paranasal or sinus infection in patients with chronic rhinitis and asthma. In summary, population studies strongly highlight a common association of disease of the upper airway, as well as the lower airway. These studies, of course, do not establish a direct pathophysiologic link.

Various studies have indicated that morphologic and physiologic parameters of both the nasal and the lower airway compartments are quite similar. Compo-

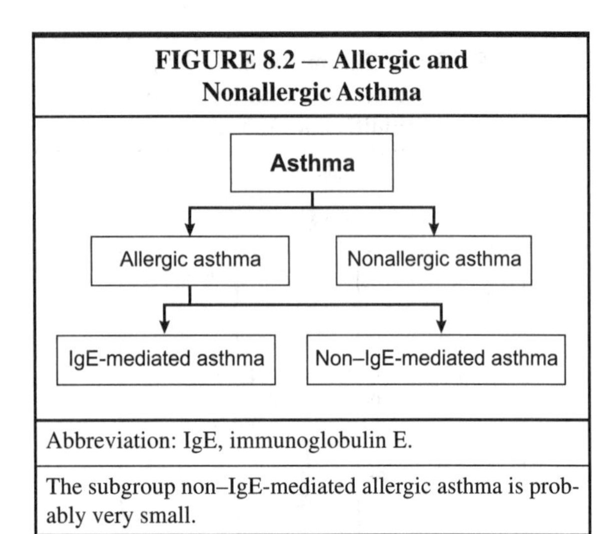

FIGURE 8.2 — Allergic and Nonallergic Asthma

Abbreviation: IgE, immunoglobulin E.

The subgroup non–IgE-mediated allergic asthma is probably very small.

sition of the cells (ie, epithelial cells, mucous glands, eosinophils, T-helper 2 [T_{H2}] lymphocytes, mast cells and basophils) and soluble immune mediators (ie, interleukin [IL]-4, 5, and 13, leukotrienes) is similar. Proinflammatory mediators, such as nitric oxide (NO), are produced in both compartments.

Experimental provocation studies have strongly established the interconnected nature of nasal and bronchial passages. Patients with seasonal allergic rhinitis (SAR) without clinical evidence of asthma often have bronchial hyperresponsiveness by methacholine provocation. Fifty percent of subjects tested during the relevant allergy season were methacholine-positive, whereas 11% to 73% were positive when tested out of season. Nasal allergen challenge with grass pollen extracts followed by sequential sampling of both nasal and bronchial mucosa indicated similar infiltration of eosinophils, IL-5–positive lymphocytes, and adhesion molecules at 24 hours in both compartments. Similarly, patients with allergic rhinitis who underwent bronchoscopic segmental allergen challenge developed increased eosinophils in the nasal mucosa as well as the systemic circulation. In summary, these data strongly indicate that provocation of either the nose or lung has a secondary effect on the other.

Several clinical studies clearly indicate that treatment of rhinitis with intranasal steroids improves bronchial symptoms, the rate of hospital admission, the number of emergency department visits for asthma exacerbation, and lower bronchial hyperreactivity, as well as lower levels for markers of inflammation, such as NO. Similarly, in patients with persistent asthma and allergic rhinitis, therapy of rhinitis with antihistamines (ie, loratadine, cetirizine) reduces nasal symptoms as well as the frequency and severity of lower respiratory symptoms. Similar data indicate that both desloratadine and montelukast are effective in reducing asthma symptoms and bronchodilator use in patients with coexistent asthma and SAR. Additional data suggest that the combination of an antihistamine and a leukotriene antagonist would be an effective approach in patients with coexistent asthma and SAR to both reduce symptoms as well as protect against bronchoconstrictor stimuli.

Omalizumab

Multiple studies have shown omalizumab (Xolair) to be effective in immunoglobulin E (IgE)-mediated allergic rhinitis. Adelroth randomized 536 patients between 12 and 75 years of age with at least a 2-year history of ragweed-induced allergic rhinitis to receive omalizumab (300 mg, 150 mg, or 50 mg) or placebo every 3 weeks (if their IgE levels were between 151 and 700 IU/mL), or every 4 weeks (if their IgE levels were between 30 and 150 IU/mL). The main outcome measures were the self-assessed daily nasal symptom-severity score, which ranged from 0 (no symptoms) to 3, and frequency of rescue antihistamine use. The nasal symptom-severity scores were significantly lower with a 300-mg dose than with placebo (0.75 vs 0.98, respectively; $P = 0.002$). Patients in the 300-mg and 150-mg groups used rescue antihistamines less frequently than patients on placebo (12% and 13% of the days for the 300-mg and 150-mg groups vs 21% of the days for patients on placebo, respectively). Had patients in all groups been required to use the same amount of oral antihistamines, the difference in symptom levels between the treatment and the placebo groups would likely have been larger.

Other data indicate significant improvement of rhinitis-specific quality of life with use of omalizumab. Additional studies have evaluated adding omalizumab to specific immunotherapy in adolescents with birch pollen– or grass pollen–induced SAR. Omalizumab used for 4 weeks in addition to specific immunotherapy significantly reduced the use of rescue medication and significantly improved allergy symptoms compared with specific immunotherapy alone. In studies involving moderate-to-severe perennial allergic rhinitis, 16 weeks of treatment with omalizumab subcutaneously every 3 to 4 weeks significantly reduced the severity of nasal and ocular symptoms, significantly reduced rescue medication usage, and significantly improved rhinoconjunctivitis-specific quality of life compared with placebo.

Only one study to date has examined the efficacy of omalizumab as an add-on therapy for patients with concomitant allergic asthma and persistent allergic rhinitis. A total of 405 patients who had suboptimal control of asthma with a stable treatment of inhaled steroids (ie, ≥400 µg budesonide) requiring more than two unscheduled visits for asthma during the past year were treated with subcutaneous omalizumab every 4 weeks. Patients treated with omalizumab experienced fewer asthma exacerbations (20.6%) than placebo-treated patients (30.1%, $P = 0.02$). Significant improvement in both Asthma Quality of Life Questionnaire and Rhinitis Quality of Life Questionnaire were seen in omalizumab-treated patients compared with placebo-treated patients. Serious adverse events were observed in 1.4% of omalizumab-treated patients and 1.5% of placebo-treated patients.

Currently, omalizumab is not approved for patients with rhinitis. However, in patients who have both rhinitis and severe difficult-to-control asthma, available data would indicate that omalizumab is an effective option. Omalizumab 150 mg to 375 mg is administered subcutaneously every 2 or 4 weeks.

9 Rhinosinusitis: Definition, Classification, and Epidemiology

Definition

Sinusitis may be defined as inflammation of the paranasal sinuses due to a variety of etiologies. More recently, *rhinosinusitis* has become the preferred term for this common clinical syndrome since inflammation of the sinuses is usually associated with concomitant disease of the nose and nasal mucosa. The most common types of rhinosinusitis are of allergic or viral etiology. Viral rhinosinusitis (VRS) usually precedes a secondary bacterial rhinosinusitis. **Table 9.1** lists the differential diagnosis of rhinosinusitis.

Classification

Most of the discussion here will be focused on community-acquired acute bacterial rhinosinusitis (ABRS) since this is a common and vexing clinical entity for the practitioner. VRS has been identified by computerized tomographic scans in approximately 90% of patients with a viral upper respiratory infection (URI) (ie, "common cold") (**Table 9.2**). A small percentage of these patients may develop a secondary bacterial infection. A typical viral URI due to organisms such as rhinovirus, coronavirus, or influenzae is hallmarked by symptoms, including:

- Sneezing
- Rhinorrhea
- Nasal congestion

TABLE 9.1 — Differential Diagnosis of Rhinosinusitis

- Infectious rhinitis
  - Viral upper respiratory tract infection
  - Bacterial rhinosinusitis
- Allergic rhinitis (seasonal or perennial)
- Nonallergic rhinitis (idiopathic rhinitis), which includes:
  - Vasomotor rhinitis
  - Eosinophilic nonallergic rhinitis (NARES)
  - Endocrine rhinitis
    - Hormonal
    - Pregnancy
    - Hypothyroidism
  - Granulomatous rhinitis (Wegener's)
- Rhinitis medicamentosa
- Anatomic deformities
- Nasal septal obstructions
- Nasal turbinate hypertrophy
- Concha bullosa of middle turbinates
- Tumors

Adapted from: Kaliner MA. *Am J Med Sci*. 1998;16:21-28.

- Postnasal drip
- Sore throat
- Cough
- Fever
- Myalgia
- Decreased sensation of smell (hyposmia/anosmia)
- Facial pressure
- Fullness of the ears.

Nasal discharge may be clear or purulent and yellow in color and still be caused by a viral infection. A typical viral URI improves within 5 to 7 days and usually largely resolves by 10 to 14 days. Bacterial superinfection or ABRS can be considered when symptoms persist beyond 10 days or worsen after 5 to 7 days.

TABLE 9.2 — Classification of Adult Rhinosinusitis

Classification	Duration	Special Notes
Acute	$\leq$4 weeks	Fever or facial pain does not constitute a suggestive history in the absence of other nasal signs or symptoms; consider acute bacterial rhinosinusitis if symptoms worsen after 5 days, if symptoms persist for >10 days, or in the presence of symptoms out of proportion to those typically associated with viral infection
Subacute	4–12 weeks	Complete resolution after effective medical therapy
Recurrent acute	$\geq$4 episodes per year, with each episode lasting $\geq$7-10 days and absence of intervening signs and symptoms of chronic rhinosinusitis	—
Chronic	$\geq$12 weeks	Facial pain does not constitute a suggestive history in the absence of other nasal signs or symptoms
Acute exacerbations of chronic	Sudden worsening of chronic rhinosinusitis, with return to baseline after treatment	—

Lanza DC, et al. *Otolaryngol Head Neck Surg*. 1997;117:S1-S7.

9

The term ABRS is used when symptoms of inflammation range from 10 days to 4 weeks; subacute bacterial rhinosinusitis is from 4 to 12 weeks, and chronic rhinosinusitis is generally defined as symptoms lasting >12 weeks. Recurring infection that resolves completely between episodes is termed recurrent ABRS.

Epidemiology

The epidemiology and financial impact of ABRS are impressive. In the United States, it is believed that the incidence of viral URIs is about two to three episodes per adult per year and as high as 6 to 8 episodes per year in children. Simple math indicates that there are probably about 1 billion episodes of viral URI per year. Some data indicate that roughly 0.5% to 2% of viral URIs are complicated by ABRS or, in other words, approximately 20 to 30 million Americans are affected each year. Primary diagnoses of rhinosinusitis lead to expenditures of approximately $3.4 billion in the United States. These data strongly indicate that ABRS is a common problem that most clinicians are likely to encounter and that it produces a great deal of suffering for patients. Clinicians need to be quite adept at and comfortable with managing this entity.

10

Rhinosinusitis: Anatomy and Pathophysiology

The sinuses develop from the nasal chamber. At birth, the maxillary and ethmoid sinuses can be identified. The overall growth of paranasal sinuses is slow for the first 6 years of life, with the original opening (ostium) remaining small. After age 6 to 7 years, the shape of the sinuses becomes irregular due to the distorting effects by the developing adjacent structures, including the other paranasal sinuses. By age 12 to 14 years, most of the sinuses have reached adult shape and almost adult size. The precise age at which growth is complete is impossible to determine. Some sinuses continue to grow even into late adulthood. The maxillary, sphenoid, and frontal sinuses are large, paired, bony chambers, whereas the anterior and posterior ethmoid sinuses consist of a labyrinth of small bony cells (**Figure 10.1**). The maxillary sinuses, the frontal sinuses, and the anterior ethmoid air cells all drain into the middle meatus beneath the middle turbinate (**Color Plate 1**). The normal middle meatus is only a few millimeters wide. The posterior ethmoids and sphenoids drain into the superior meatus and sphenoethmoidal recess.

The evolutionary function of the paranasal sinuses is unclear and it has been suggested historically that these structures:

- Are important in warming and humidifying inspired air
- Are important for a resonance quality to the voice
- May be important to reduce the bony mass and weight of the skull.

FIGURE 10.1 — Schematic Drawing (Coronal View) of Nose and Paranasal Sinuses

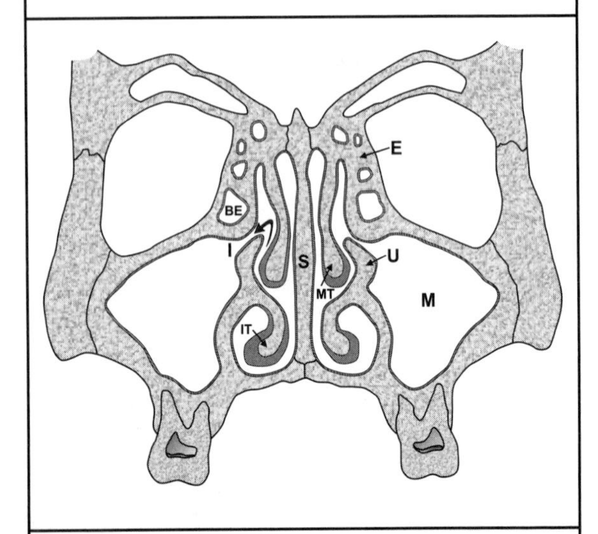

Abbreviations: BE, bulla ethmoidalis; E, ethmoids; I, maxillary sinus infundibulum; IT, inferior turbinate; M, maxillary sinus; MT, middle turbinate; S, nasal septum; U, uncinate process; curved arrow: hiatus semilunaris

Adapted from: Levine HL, May M. *Endoscopic Sinus Surgery*. New York: Thieme Medical Publishers, Inc; 1993:247.

Newer research has demonstrated that the paranasal sinuses are a large reservoir for nitric oxide (NO), which improves mucociliary function. NO has been shown to be bacteriostatic as well as antiviral and to improve lung function. Acute or chronic inflammation of the nose and paranasal sinuses leads to increased NO production.

Viral rhinitis due to pathogens such as rhinovirus and coronavirus usually precede the development of a secondary acute bacterial rhinosinusitis (ABRS). Infection with the upper respiratory tract viruses leads to generalized mucosal edema, up-regulation of

COLOR PLATE 1
View of Lateral Wall of Nose Demonstrating Relationships of Sinus Openings

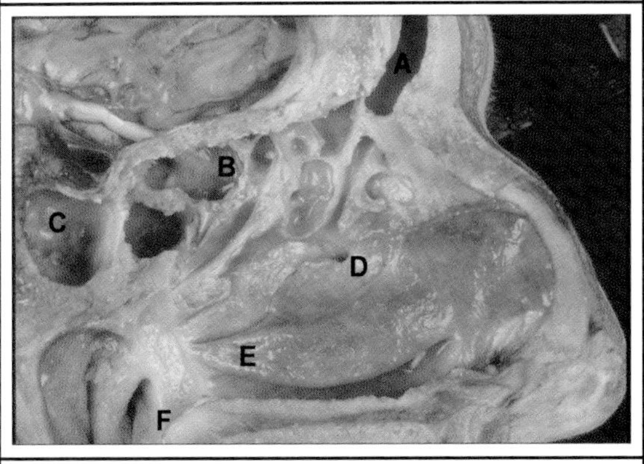

(A) frontal sinus; *(B)* ethmoid sinus; *(C)* sphenoid sinus; *(D)* opening to maxillary sinus; *(E)* inferior turbinate; *(F)* eustachian tube

Courtesy of JB Anon, MD.

COLOR PLATE 2
Nasal Endoscopic Image of Right Lateral Nasal Wall

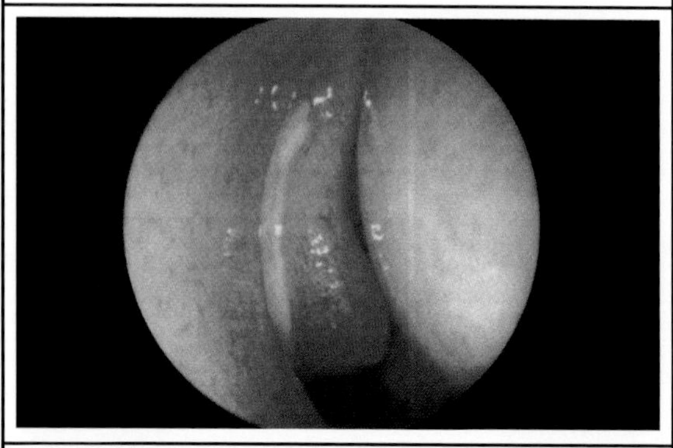

Nasal endoscopic image of right lateral nasal wall with mucopurulent drainage in the middle meatus under the middle turbinate indicating acute baterial rhinosinusitis.

Courtesy JA Hadley, MD.

COLOR PLATE 3
Nasal Examination and Culture

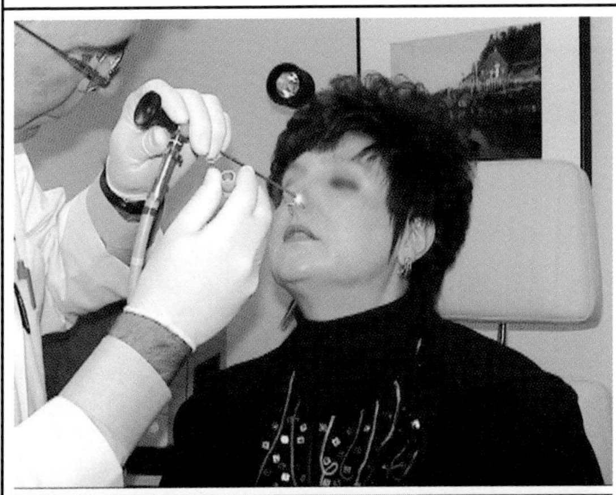

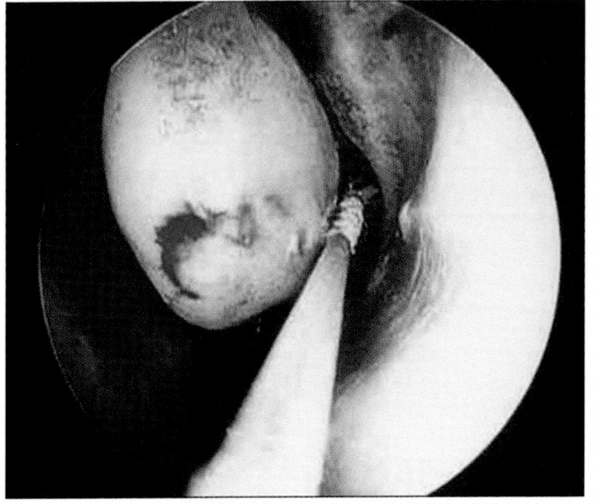

(Top) Physician performing nasal endoscopy with culture on patient. *(Bottom)* Culturing pus in the nose.

Courtesy JA Hadley, MD.

COLOR PLATE 4
Radiograph Demonstrating Bilateral Air-Fluid Levels of Maxillary Sinuses

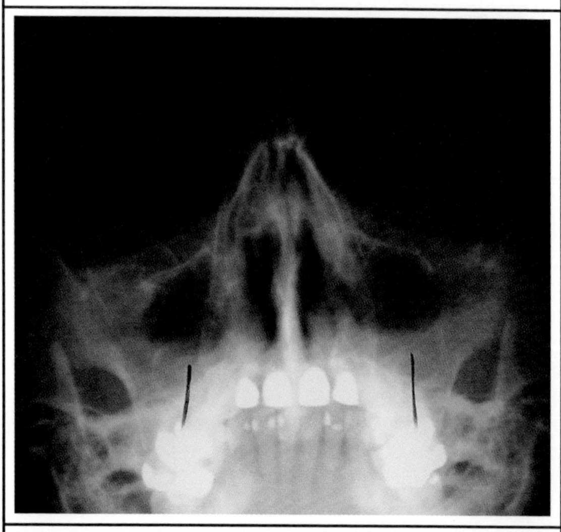

Black lines are pointing to fluid.

Courtesy JA Hadley, MD.

COLOR PLATE 5
Plain Radiograph of Right Maxillary Opacification

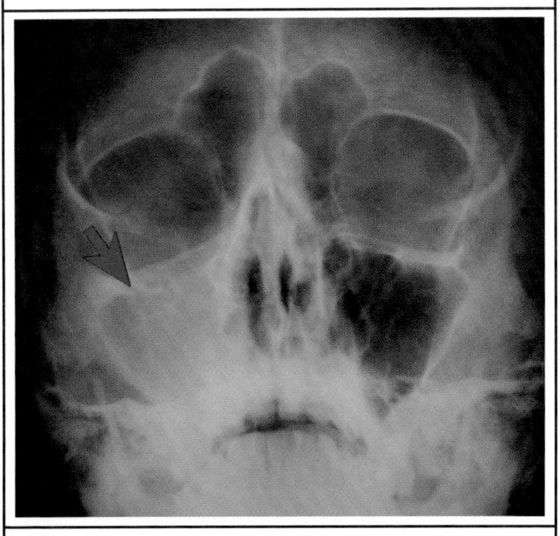

Acute right maxillary sinusitis with plain radiograph showing complete opacification of right sinus.

Courtesy JA Hadley, MD.

COLOR PLATE 6
Antrochoanal Polyp

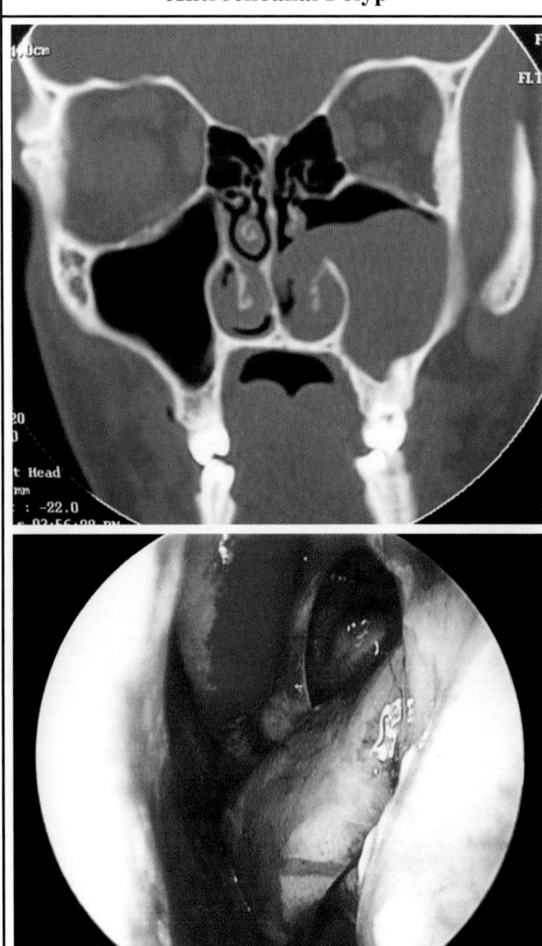

Large left antrochoanal polyp blocking left nasal cavity.

Courtesy JA Hadley, MD.

COLOR PLATE 7
Computed Tomography Scans of Various Degrees of Acute and Chronic Rhinosinusitis

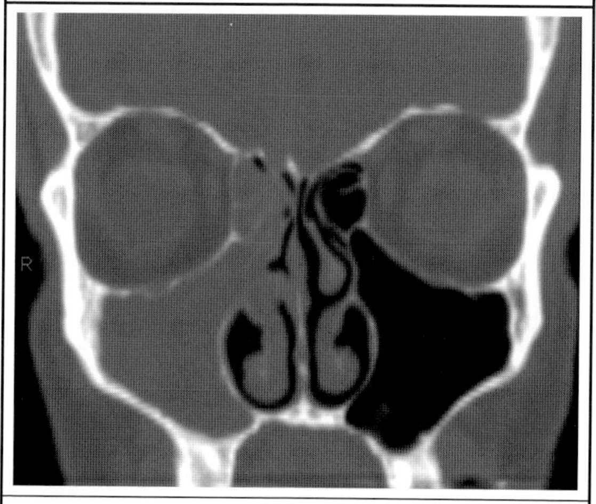

Computed tomography (CT) scan shows complete opacification of the right maxillary sinus.

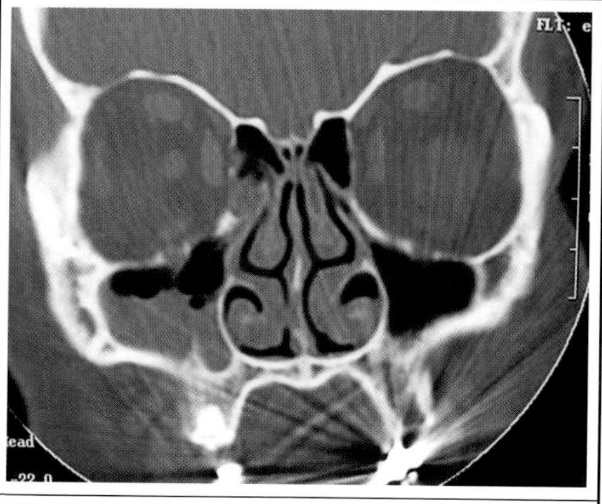

CT scan shows acute rhinosinusitis and air-fluid level of right maxillary sinus with obstruction of the osteomeatal area.

Continued

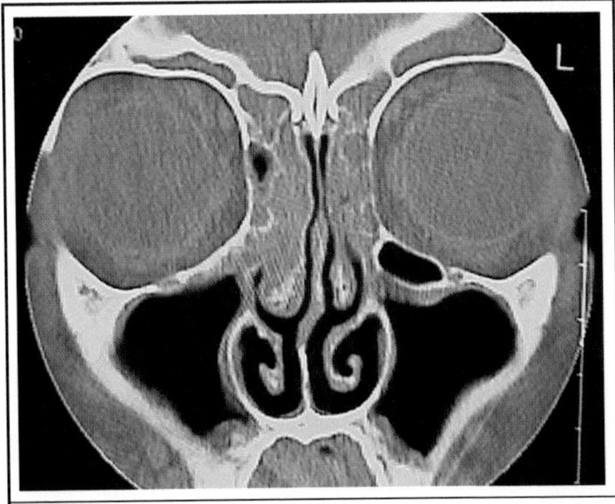

CT scan shows both ethmoid sinuses are opacified but little to no maxillary sinusitis.

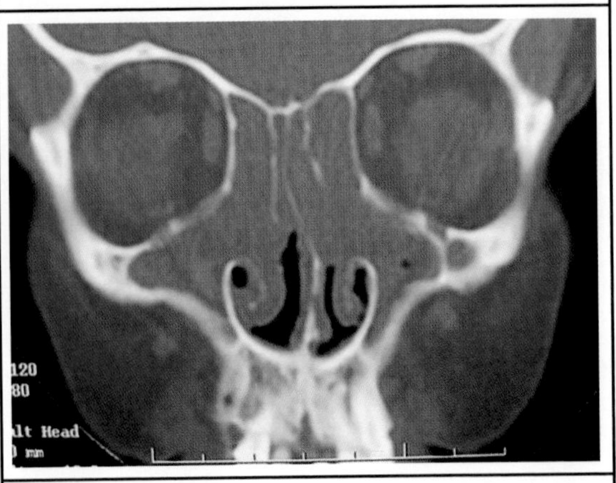

CT scan shows complete opacification of all the sinuses.

Courtesy JA Hadley, MD.

COLOR PLATE 8
Computed Tomography Scan Demonstrating Air-Fluid Levels

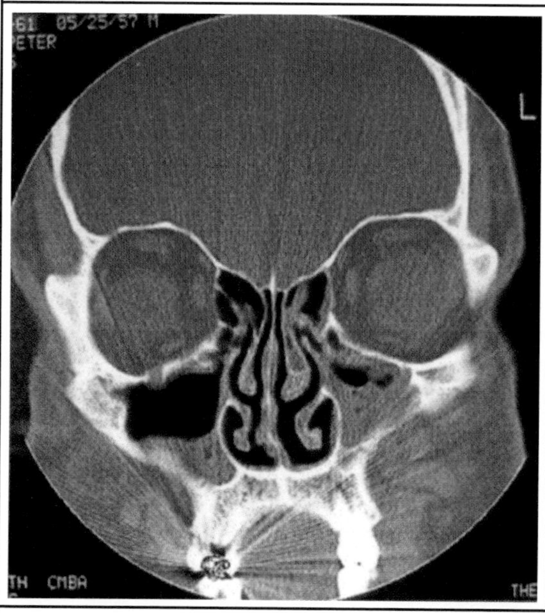

Computed tomography (CT) scan demonstrating air-fluid levels due to acute infection within the maxillary sinuses.

Courtesy JA Hadley, MD.

COLOR PLATE 9
Computed Tomography Scan Demonstrating Air-Fluid Levels and Opacification

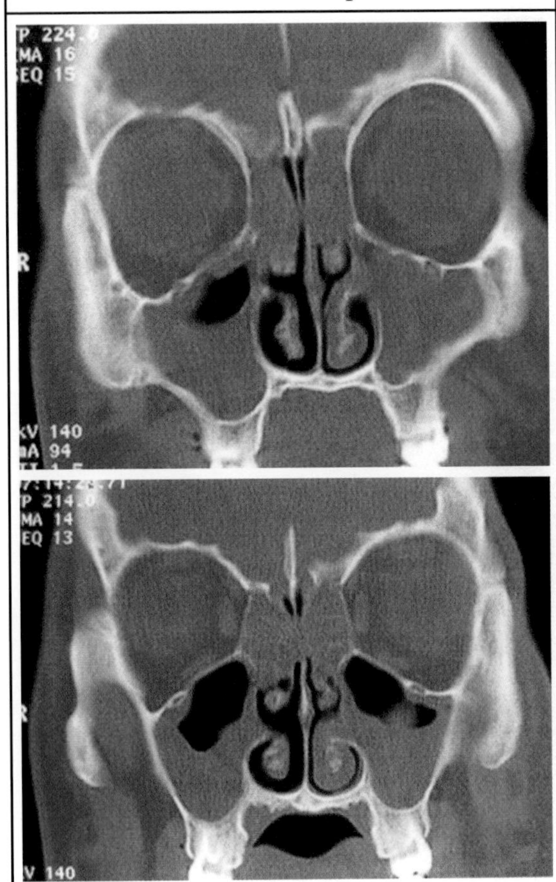

Computed tomography (CT) scan demonstrates air-fluid levels and opacification of maxillary sinuses, but normal ethmoids.

Courtesy JA Hadley, MD.

COLOR PLATES 10
Nasal Endoscopic Examination Demonstrating Thick Nasal Secretions

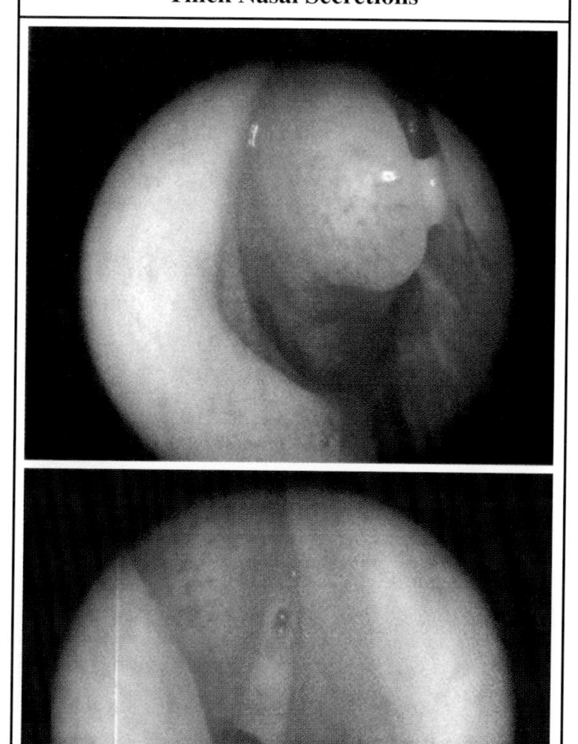

Nasal endoscopic examination demonstrating thick nasal secretions from both drainage pathways.

Courtesy JA Hadley, MD.

COLOR PLATE 11
Three Days After Initial Symptoms of Left Nasal Congestion and Left Facial Pain

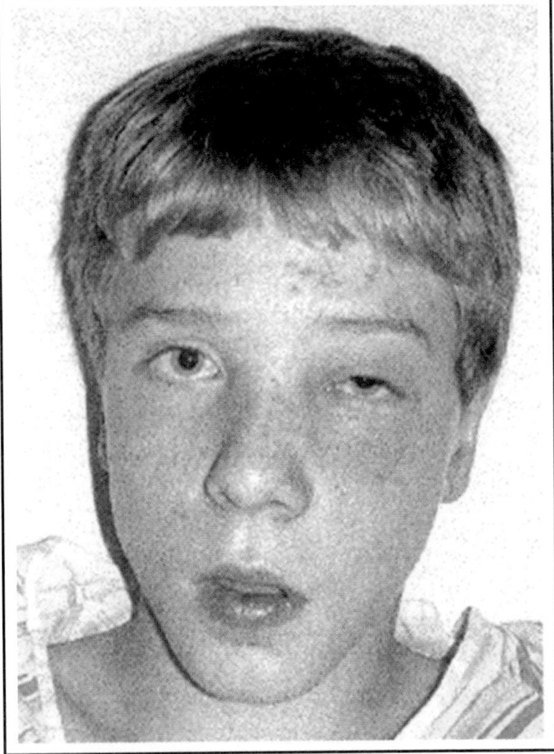

Thirteen-year-old male 3 days after initial symptoms of left nasal congestion and left nasal pain.

Courtesy JA Hadley, MD.

proinflammatory mediators, and changes in binding sites, whereby bacteria may attach more readily to nasal and sinus mucosa. Ordinarily, the sinuses are a sterile environment. However, the nasopharynx and lateral nose are colonized by a variety of organisms that are etiologically important in sinus disease. A variety of physical factors — one of which is nose blowing — help facilitate the translocation of bacteria into the sinus cavities.

Nasal endoscopy with Gram's stain has about an 85% concordance with what some consider the gold standard to assess the presence of bacteria within the sinuses: needle aspiration of the maxillary sinus. The maxillary sinus may be approached either through a sublabial or inferior meatal puncture.

The most common bacterial isolates recovered from the maxillary sinuses of patients with ABRS are *Streptococcus pneumoniae*, *Haemophilus influenzae,* other streptococcal species, and *Moraxella catarrhalis*. A review of sinus aspiration studies performed in adults with ABRS finds that *S pneumoniae* is isolated in approximately 20% to 43%, *H influenzae* in 22% to 35%, and *M catarrhalis* in 2% to 10% of aspirates (**Figure 10.2**). In children with ABRS, *S pneumoniae* is identified in approximately 35% to 42%, while *H influenzae* and *M catarrhalis* each are recovered from about 21% to 28% of aspirates (**Figure 10.3**). Other bacterial isolates found in patients with ABRS include *Streptococcus pyogenes, Staphylococcus aureus,* and anaerobes.

It is interesting to note that the same bacterial pathogens are important in ABRS in several parts of the world. In addition, the spectrum of pathogens has not changed over the past 40 years. Importantly, the primary change has been the increased use of antibiotics and, therefore, the emergence of antibiotic resistance in these organisms.

FIGURE 10.2 — Ranges of Prevalence of the Major Pathogens Associated With Acute Bacterial Rhinosinusitis in Adults

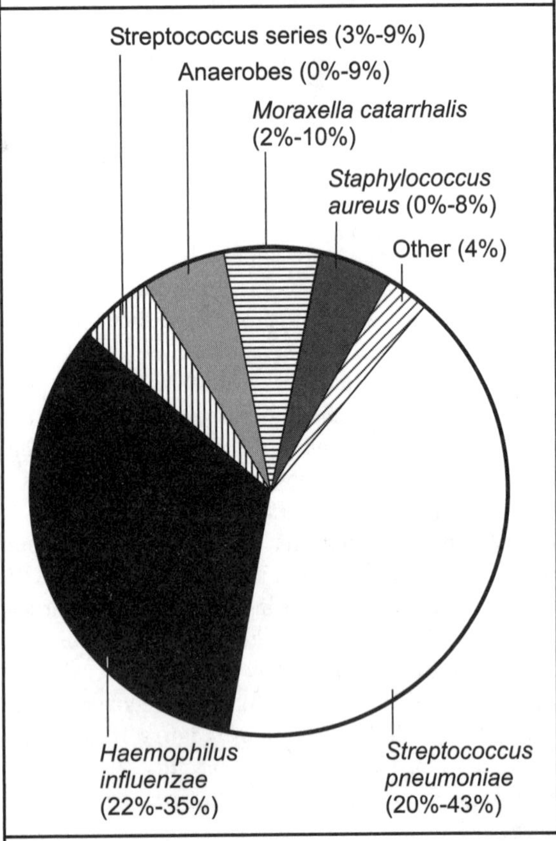

Sinus and Allergy Health Partnership. *Otolaryngol Head Neck Surg*. 2004;130(suppl):S12.

Antibiotic resistance may occur by one of several mechanisms. One mechanism is by the production of antibiotic-inactivating enzymes; the best example is the production of β-lactamase (**Figure 10.4**). These are enzymes that hydrolyze the amide bond of the β-lactam

FIGURE 10.3 — Microbiology of Acute Bacterial Rhinosinusitis in Children

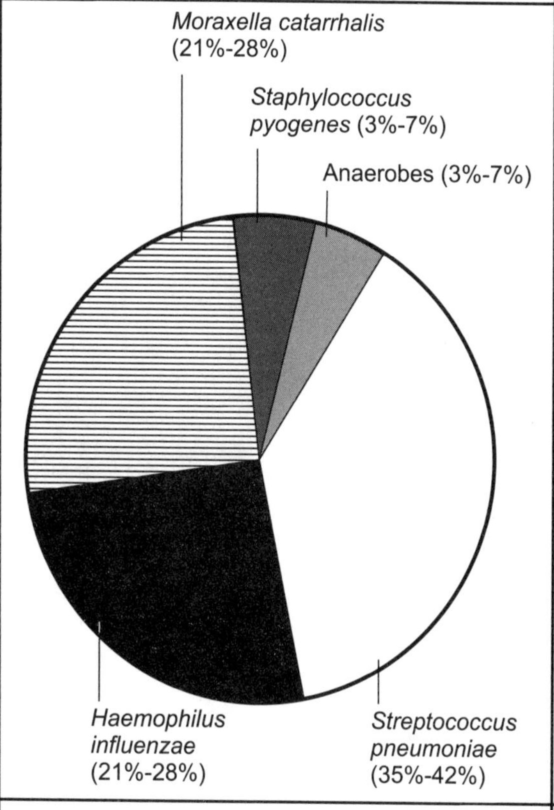

Sinus and Allergy Health Partnership. *Otolaryngol Head Neck Surg*. 2004;130(suppl):S12.

10

ring, resulting in inactivation. Important β-lactamase–producing bacteria include *H influenzae* and *M catarrhalis*. The second important mechanism of bacterial resistance is the alteration of the antimicrobial target or binding site in the bacteria. A well-characterized example of this mechanism is *S pneumoniae*, where resistance to β-lactams develops as a stepwise

FIGURE 10.4 — Antibiotic Inactivation by β-Lactamases Such as Those of *Haemophilus influenzae* and *Moraxella catarrhalis*

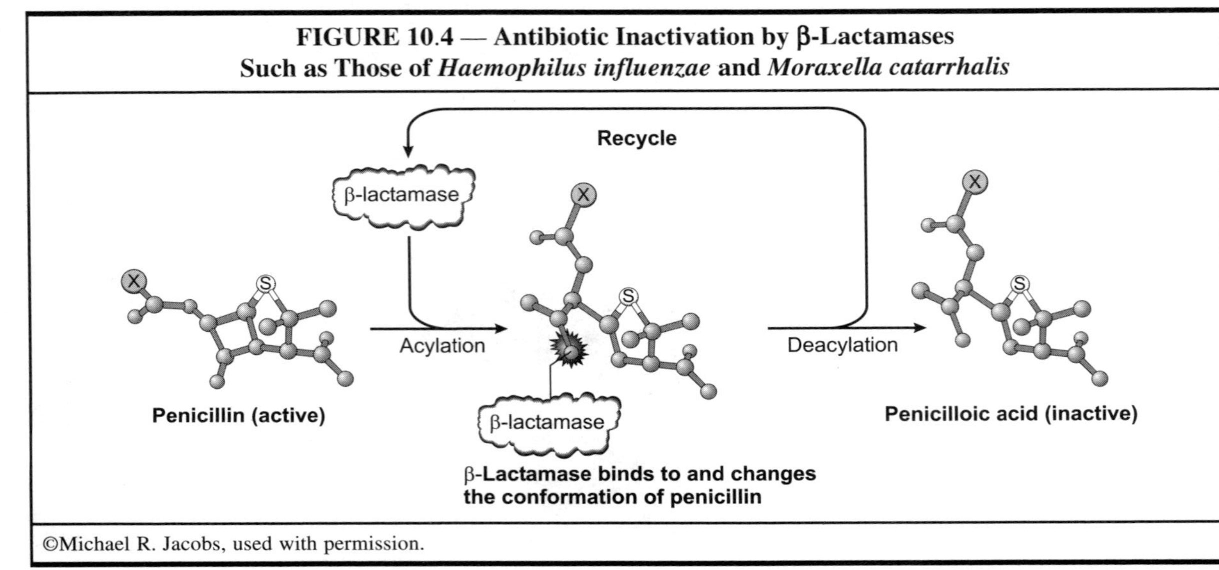

alteration of penicillin-binding proteins (PBPs) that leads to a decrease in the binding affinity of the β-lactams. PBP 1a, 2b, 2x alterations are responsible for most of the resistance in *S pneumoniae*. Efflux mechanisms pump the antibiotic out of the cell before the antibiotic can attach to a receptor, such as with macrolides and fluoroquinolones.

In the laboratory setting, *S pneumoniae* is considered susceptible to penicillin if the minimum inhibitory concentration (MIC) is ≤0.06 mg/mL. Intermediate and resistant strains have MICs of 0.12–1.0 and 2.0 mg/mL, respectively. Penicillin–nonsusceptible *S pneumoniae* emerged in the late 1980s and represents a major problem in some communities. **Figure 10.5** and **Figure 10.6** indicate the prevalence of penicillin-resistant *S pneumoniae* and β-lactamase–producing *H influenzae* in the United States. Current surveillance studies demonstrate that about 30% of *S pneumoniae* isolates are penicillin resistant. An important observation is that many of the penicillin–nonsusceptible isolates have a fairly high incidence of resistance to trimethoprim/sulfamethoxazole (TMP/SMX), macrolides, clindamycin, and doxycycline (**Table 10.1**). Only 2% of the isolates of *S pneumoniae* are resistant to the respiratory fluoroquinolones. **Table 10.2** summarizes antimicrobial agents stratified by pharmacodynamic profile against *S pneumoniae* and *H influenzae*.

Primary mechanism of resistance for isolates of *H influenzae* and *M catarrhalis* is through β-lactamase production (**Table 10.3** and **Figure 10.7**). Over the decade from 1986 to 1998, the percent of β-lactamase–producing *H influenzae* has increased from 10% to about 40% in the United States. Macrolides and ketolides have reduced activity against *H influenza*. About 24% of isolates of *H influenzae* were resistant to TMP/SMX and none were fluoroquinolone-resistant. Also, the β-lactams amoxicillin/clavulanate, cefdinir, and cefpodoxime proxetil are effective against

FIGURE 10.5 — Prevalence of Nonsusceptible Intermediate and Resistant *Streptococcus pneumoniae* to Penicillin

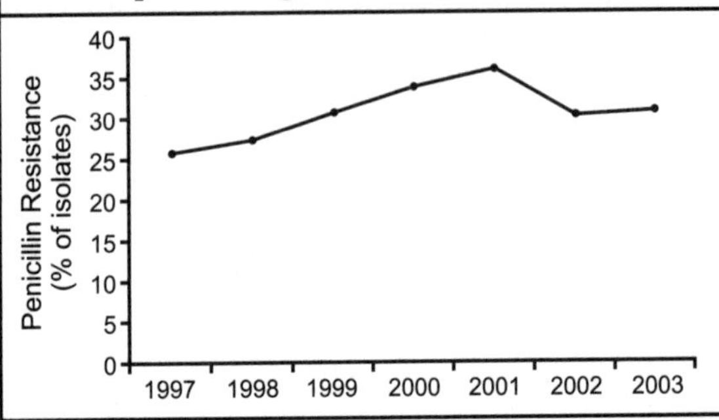

Prevalence of nonsusceptible intermediate and resistant *S pneumoniae* to penicillin has been increasing over the past decade in the United States. Percentages ranged from 25% to 50%, depending on the surveillance study used in 1997 to 2003.

Sinus and Allergy Health Partnership. *Otolaryngol Head Neck Surg*. 2004;130(suppl):S15.

FIGURE 10.6 — Prevalence of β-Lactamase Production by *Haemophilus influenzae* in the United States From 1997 to 2003

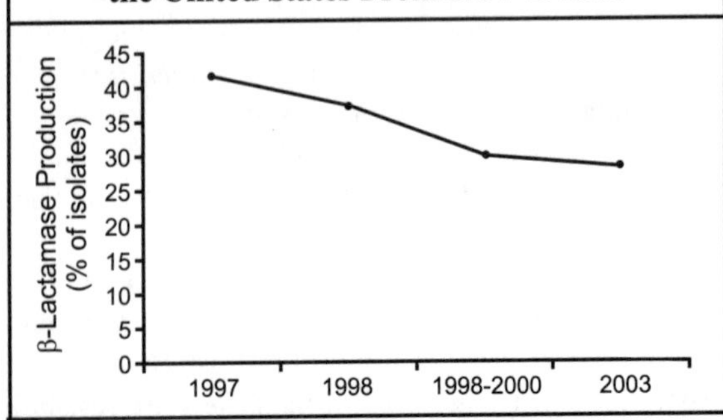

Sinus and Allergy Health Partnership. *Otolaryngol Head Neck Surg*. 2004;130(suppl):S16.

TABLE 10.1 — Prevalence of Cross-Resistance Between Penicillin and Various Antibiotic Classes Among Strains of Penicillin–Nonsusceptible Strains of *Streptococcus pneumoniae*

	% of Strains Resistant			
Class/Agent	**Pen-S**	**Pen-I**	**Pen-R**	**All**
Macrolides	6	49	76	32
Clindamycin	1	14	28	10
TMP/SMX	14	57	91	43
Doxycycline	4	25	55	22

Abbreviations: MIC, minimum inhibitory concentration; Pen-I, penicillin–intermediate (penicillin MIC 0.12 mg/mL to 1 mg/mL); Pen-R, penicillin–resistant (penicillin MIC ≥2 mg/mL); Pen-S, penicillin–susceptible (penicillin MIC ≤0.06 mg/mL); TMP/SMX, trimethoprim/sulfamethoxazole.

Jacobs MR. *Pediatr Infect Dis J.* 2003;22(suppl 8):S109-S119; Jacobs MR et al. *Clin Lab Med.* 2004;24:419-453.

β-lactamase–producing *H influenzae*. The prevalence of β-lactamase–producing isolates of *M catarrhalis* is close to 100% in the United States. Also, >90% of the isolates are resistant to TMP/SMX. However, all the isolates are susceptible to amoxicillin/clavulanate, cefixime, cefdinir, telithromycin, fluoroquinolones, and macrolides/azalides.

TABLE 10.2 — Antimicrobial Agents Stratified by Pharmacodynamic Profile Against *Streptococcus pneumoniae* and *Haemophilus influenzae*

Antimicrobial Agent	Achieves Pharmacodynamic Target*				
	S pneumoniae			*H influenzae*	
	Penicillin-susceptible	Penicillin-intermediate	Penicillin-resistant	β-Lactamase–negative	β-Lactamase–positive
β-Lactams					
Amoxicillin[†]	✓	✓	✓	✓	
Amoxicillin/clavulanate[†]	✓	✓	✓	✓	✓
Cefdinir	✓	±		✓	✓
Cefpodoxime	✓	✓		✓	✓
Ceftriaxone	✓	✓	✓	✓	✓
Cefuroxime	✓	✓		✓	✓
Folate Inhibitors					
TMP/SMX	✓	±		✓	✓
Ketolides					
Telithromycin	✓	✓	✓	±	±
Macrolides					
Azithromycin	✓	±		±	±

Clarithromycin	✓	±		±	±
Erythromycin	✓	±			
Fluoroquinolones					
Gatifloxacin	✓	✓	✓	✓	✓
Gemifloxacin	✓	✓	✓	✓	✓
Levofloxacin	✓	✓	✓	✓	✓
Moxifloxacin	✓	✓	✓	✓	✓
Tetracyclines					
Doxycycline	✓	✓	±		

Abbreviations: AUC, area under the curve; MIC, minimum inhibitory concentration; TMP/SMX, trimethoprim/sulfamethoxazole.

Key: ✓, Adequate pharmacodynamic profile using conventional dosing in patients with normal renal and hepatic function; ±, borderline pharmacodynamic profile using conventional dosing in patients with normal renal and hepatic function.

* β-Lactams and macrolides: T > MIC >40% of the dosing interval. Fluoroquinolones: 24-h AUC/MIC ratio >100-125 for *H influenzae* and >30-50 for *S pneumoniae*.

† High-dose amoxicillin.

Modified from Sinus and Allergy Health Partnership. *Otolaryngol Head Neck Surg*. 2004;130(suppl):S1-S45.

TABLE 10.3 — Mechanisms of Action of Commonly Used Antimicrobials for Community-Acquired Respiratory Tract Infections

Target	Examples
Cell-wall–active agents	β-Lactams (penicillins, cephalosporins)
Protein synthesis inhibitors (ribosome)	Macrolides, lincosamides (eg, clindamycin), tetracyclines (eg, tetracycline, doxycycline), ketolides
DNA replication inhibitors	Fluoroquinolones
Folic acid metabolism inhibitors	Trimethoprim/ sulfamethoxazole

Jacobs MR, et al. *Clin Lab Med*. 2004;24:419-453.

FIGURE 10.7 — Major Antibiotic Targets of the Prokaryotic Cell

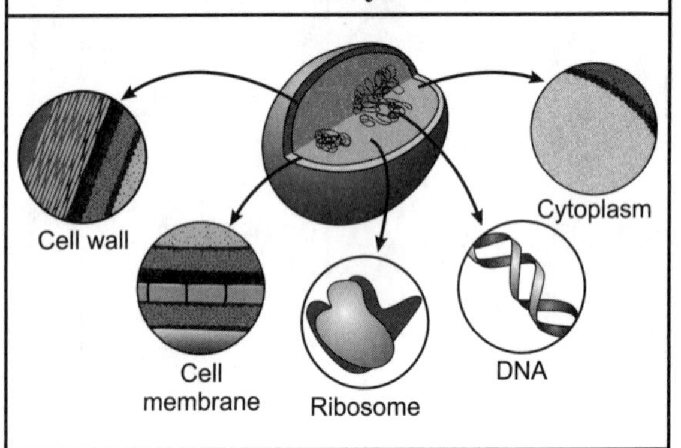

The major antibiotic targets of the prokaryotic cell, including cell wall, cell membrane, ribosome, DNA, and cytoplasm.

11 Rhinosinusitis: Diagnosis

Acute bacterial rhinosinusitis (ABRS) is a clinical diagnosis that can be suspected based on a constellation of symptoms due to a viral upper respiratory tract infection that persist for 10 days or more *or* symptoms that worsen after 5 to 7 days. Symptoms may include:

- Persistent nasal drainage or congestion
- Postnasal drip
- Fever
- Cough
- Facial pain/pressure
- Maxillary dental pain
- Hyposmia/anosmia
- Ear fullness/pressure
- Fatigue.

Overall, the accuracy of signs and symptoms in diagnosing ABRS is suboptimal. The change in the color of the nasal drainage is generally believed not to be a marker for bacterial infection, although further research in this area is needed. Maxillary toothache has high specificity (93%) but a sensitivity of only 18%. Physical examination of patients with ABRS is generally limited because paranasal sinuses are largely hidden within the skull and cannot be directly examined. Sinus tenderness on exam has a sensitivity of 45% and a specificity of 65%. Facial pain is not a common complaint in children. Facial tenderness is an unreliable sign in small children.

Anterior rhinoscopy with a topical decongestant can detect purulent secretions within the anterior nose, and the position of the nasal septum and allows examination of the mucosa of the inferior turbinate. Posterior rhinoscopy performed with a mirror may reveal pus flowing over the posterior end of the anterior turbinate. The maxillary sinus is frequently involved in ABRS and purulent secretions drain into the middle meatus. Nasal endoscopy may establish a more definitive diagnosis of ABRS if purulent discharge is observed streaming from beneath the middle or superior turbinate (**Color Plate 2**). However, endoscopy is not generally necessary for uncomplicated cases of ABRS. Some investigators obtain endoscopic sinonasal cultures to assist in the antibiotic selection (**Color Plate 3**). Transillumination of the maxillary and frontal sinuses has limited utility since it does not distinguish bacterial from viral infection and it suffers from interobserver variability.

There is usually not a need for imaging studies in the initial management of ABRS. However, in patients with recurrent, persistent, or chronic rhinosinusitis, or if there is a complication such as an orbital infection, these studies are invaluable. Sinus imaging may be performed with plain radiographs, computed tomography (CT), and magnetic resonance imaging. Plain radiographs of the sinuses are still probably performed most often, although CT is increasingly being used as the initial imaging study. Plain films are most accurate for imaging the maxillary and frontal sinuses, and they are poor for the ethmoids. A recent meta-analysis showed that positive plain films of the sinuses have moderate sensitivity (76%) and specificity (79%) compared with maxillary sinus puncture. In adults, plain films of the sinuses have been shown to correlate with positive microbiology obtained from antral puncture in about 50% of patients. The best radiographic findings are air-fluid levels or near-complete or complete opacification (**Color Plate 4** and **Color Plate 5**). A negative plain film radiograph is a reasonable indication the patient does not have ABRS. The American Academy of Pediatrics consensus committee has recommended that imaging studies are not necessary to confirm a diagnosis of clinical rhinosinusitis in children <6 years of age.

Plain films are fraught with the limitation of not being able to evaluate the ostiomeatal complex, inability to show the extent of mucosal inflammation, and inability to visualize ethmoid air cells. **Figure 11.1** shows acute maxillary sinusitis with air-fluid level.

Computed tomography images of the paranasal sinuses provide far more detail of the sinus anatomy than plain films (**Figure 11.2** shows simple CT of normal sinuses [axial views]). A limited CT of the sinuses that includes four noncontiguous cuts in either the coronal and/or axial plane is about the same cost as a plain film sinus series with considerably less radiation exposure. Unfortunately, CT of the sinuses in patients with acute viral rhinitis might identify a variety of abnormalities in 87% of the patients, most of whom may not subsequently progress to ABRS. In general, CT studies of the sinuses can be performed in the following clinical situations:

- Nonresolving disease
- Complications or impending complications of the disease
- Recurrent rhinosinusitis
- Chronic rhinosinusitis
- Diffuse nasal polyposis
- Mucoceles
- Evaluation of possible neoplastic disease.

Some factors may predispose to development of ABRS, such as anatomical nasal septal deviation. **Figure 11.3** shows a coronal view of nasal septal deviation, and **Figure 11.4** shows a septal spur. A nice example of a large left maxillary polyp is shown in **Figure 11.5**. **Color Plate 6** shows an antrochoanal

FIGURE 11.1 — Plain Radiograph of Left Maxillary Air-Fluid Level

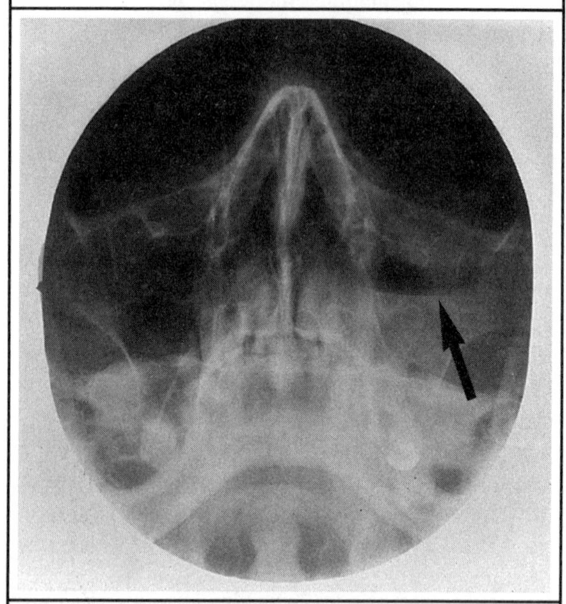

Acute left maxillary sinusitis with plain radiograph showing air-fluid level *(arrow)*.

polyp. **Figure 11.6** shows acute sinusitis. **Color Plate 7** shows CT scans of various degrees of acute and chronic rhinitis.

In general, CT imaging should be delayed during the acute phase of sinusitis until after aggressive therapy, which might include antibiotics and topical vasoconstrictor therapy. Resolution of the secondary inflammatory changes is likely to give a more accurate view of the extent of the mucosal disease as well as the ostiomeatal complex.

FIGURE 11.2 — Simple Computed Tomography of Normal Paranasal Sinuses

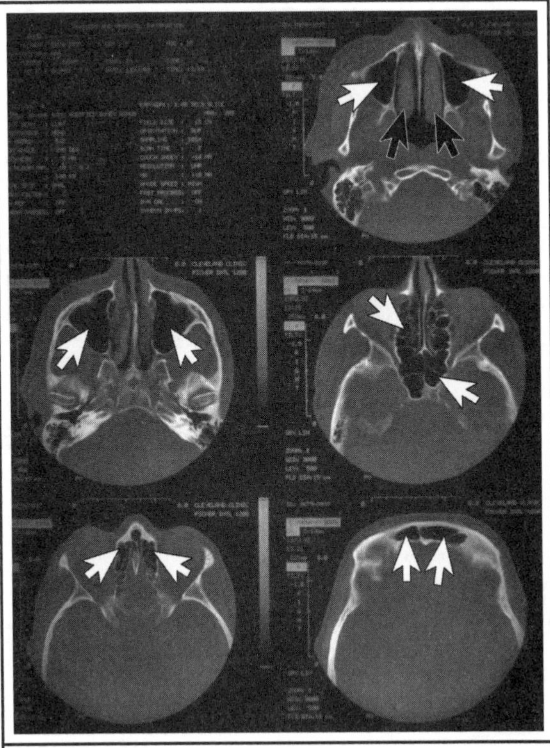

Axial views of the sinuses show: *(Top right)* Clear maxillary sinuses (white arrows) and large inferior turbinates (black arrows). *(Center left)* Clear maxillary sinuses (arrows) and a portion of the middle turbinate. *(Center right)* Clear ethmoid and sphenoid sinuses (arrows). *(Bottom left)* Clear ethmoid sinuses (arrows). *(Bottom right)* Clear frontal sinuses (arrows).

11

FIGURE 11.3 — Simple Computed Tomography of Deviated Septum

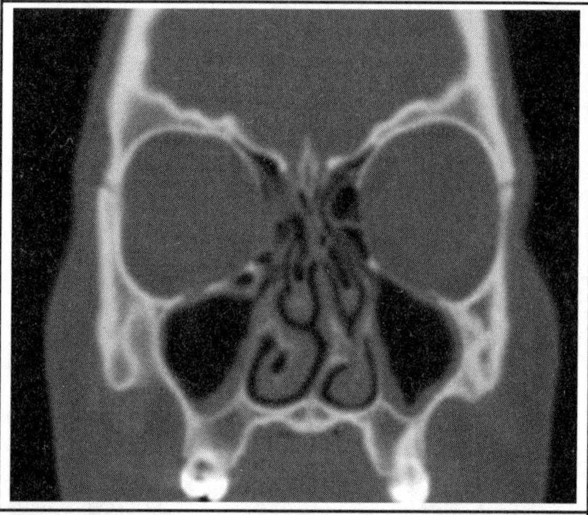

This coronal view of the sinuses reveals a nasal septum deviated to the left with minimal thickening of maxillary sinus mucosa.

Courtesy JA Hadley, MD.

FIGURE 11.4 — Simple Computed Tomography of Septal Spur

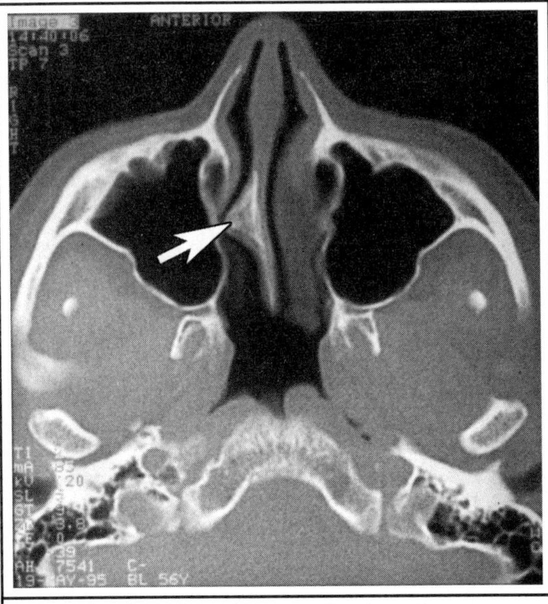

This axial view of the sinus reveals a largy bony spur on the septum *(arrow)*.

FIGURE 11.5 — Simple Computed Tomography of Left Maxillary Polyp

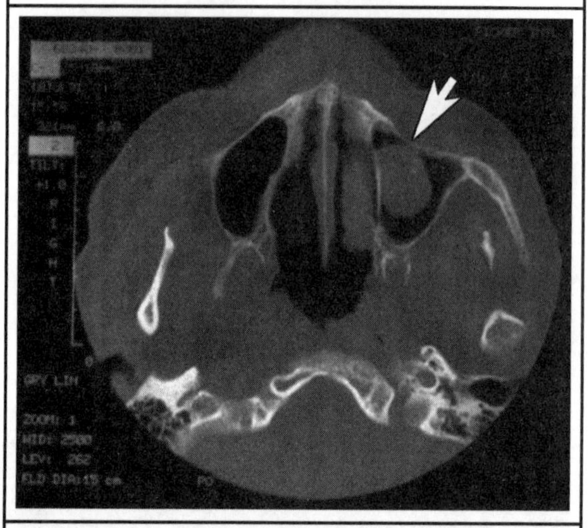

This axial view of the sinus reveals a large left maxillary polyp without evidence of sinus inflammation.

FIGURE 11.6 — Simple Computed Tomography of Bilateral Sinusitis

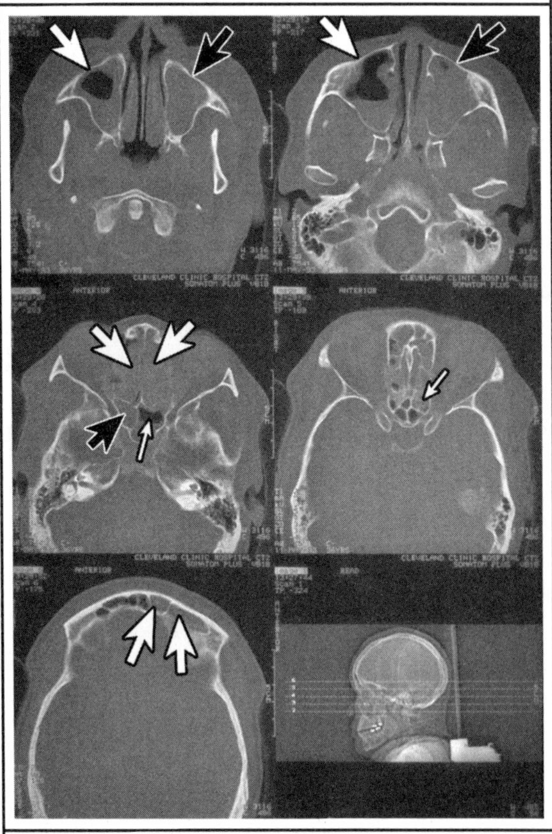

Axial views of the sinuses show: *(Top left)* Reveals an air-fluid level in the right maxillary sinus (white arrow) and opacification of the left (black arrow). *(Center left)* Shows opacification of the ethmoid sinuses (large white arrows) and the right sphenoid sinus (black arrow). *(Center left & right)* An air-fluid level in the left sphenoid sinus (small arrow). *(Bottom left)* Left frontal sinuses are seen to be opacified (arrows).

12 Acute Bacterial Rhinosinusitis: Pharmacologic Therapy

A typical viral upper respiratory infection (URI) improves within 5 to 7 days and is usually resolved by 10 days. During this initial period, symptomatic supportive care may include an antipyretic agent, decongestants (oral or topical), and hydration. Frequently patients contact the health care provider seeking an antibiotic. The Centers for Disease Control and Prevention has developed the **Get Smart** program (http://www.cdc.gov/drugresistance/community). This program and its website have pages of educational information and downloadable teaching aids to help the clinician explain why antibiotics do not work for viral disease.

When a bacterial superinfection or acute bacterial rhinosinusitis (ABRS) is suspected, it is appropriate to treat with an oral antibiotic. **Table 12.1** summarizes the available antibiotics and doses for ABRS. Empiric antibiotic therapy has changed over the past few years as resistance has emerged and as the science of understanding antibiotics (pharmacokinetics/pharmacodynamics [PK/PD]) has evolved. Antimicrobial treatment guidelines for ABRS in adults are shown in **Figure 12.1**. **Table 12.2** and **Table 12.3** summarize recent guidelines for antimicrobial treatment for adults and children with ABRS. The recommended antibiotic is based on a number of issues such as:

- Severity of the patient's illness (what is an acceptable possible failure rate for the clinician)
- Prior recent antibiotic exposure

TABLE 12.1 — Antimicrobial Agents for Acute Bacterial Rhinosinusitis

Generic Name	Trade Name	Typical Adult Dosage Regimen	Typical Pediatric Dosage Regimen	Available Dosage (mg)
β-Lactams				
Amoxicillin	Amoxil, generics	875 mg bid × 10 d	>3 mo: 45 mg/kg/d given q12h × 10 d	250, 500, 875*
Amoxicillin/ clavulanate	Augmentin	500-2000 mg bid × 10 d	≥12 wks: 45 mg/kg given q12h × 10 d	250/125, 500/125, 875/125*
	Augmentin ES-600	N/A	90 mg/kg/d divided q12h × 10 d	600 mg/5mL
	Augmentin XR	2000/125 mg bid × 10 d	N/A	1000/62.5
Cefdinir	Omnicef	300 mg bid × 10 d or 600 mg qd × 10 d	6 mo–12 yrs: 7 mg/kg q12h or 14 mg/kg q24h × 10 d	125, 250, 300*
Cefpodoxime	Vantin	200 mg bid × 10 d	2 mo–11 yrs: 5 mg/ kg/d given q12h × 10 d	100, 200*
Ceftin	Cefuroxime	250 mg bid × 10 d	3 mo–12 yrs: 15 mg/kg bid × 10 d	125, 250, 500*

Ceftriaxone	Rocephin	1-2 g IM qd × 3-10 d	50 mg/kg IM × 3 d (minimum)	500, 1 g, 2 g
Folate Inhibitors				
TMP/SMX	Bactrim, Septra	160/800 bid × 10 d	≥2 mo: 4 mg/kg TMP and 20 mg/kg SMX given q12h × 10 d	80/400, 160/800 (DS)*
Macrolides/Azalides/ Ketolides				
Azithromycin	Zithromax	500 mg qd × 3 d	≥6 mo: 10 mg/kg qd × 3 d	250, 500*
Clarithromycin	Biaxin	500 mg q12h × 14 d	≥6 mo: 7.5 mg/kg given q12h × 10 d	250, 500*
	Biaxin XL	1000 mg qd × 14 d	N/A	500
Clindamycin	Cleocin	150-300 mg q6h × 10 d	Birth–16 yrs: 8-16 mg/kg/d × 10 d	75, 150, 300*
Telithromycin	Ketek	800 qd × 5 d	N/A	400

Continued

Generic Name	Trade Name	Typical Adult Dosage Regimen	Typical Pediatric Dosage Regimen	Available Dosage (mg)
Respiratory Quinolones				
Gatifloxacin	Tequin	400 mg qd × 10 d	N/A	200, 400
Gemifloxacin	Factive	320 mg qd × 10 d	N/A	320
Levofloxacin	Levaquin	500-750 mg qd × 10 d	N/A	500, 750
Moxifloxacin	Avelox	400 mg qd × 10 d	N/A	400
Tetracyclines				
Doxycycline	Vibramycin, others	100 mg qd given q12h × 10 d	≥8 yrs; ≤100 lbs: 1 mg/lb bid on day 1, then 1 mg/lb or 0.5 mg/lb bid × 10 d	50, 75, 100*

Abbreviations: DS, double strength; N/A, not approved for use; TMP/SMX, trimethoprim/sulfamethoxazole.

This table provides typical dosage regimens; see text for full discussion.

* Some dosages are also available in suspension form.

- Odds of a specific bacteria being the culprit
- Resistance rates
- Rates of self resolution
- PK/PD profile of the prescribed antibiotic.

These data are analyzed by the Poole Therapeutic Outcome Model.

Pharmacologic Therapy for Adults

Recommendations for initial therapy for adult patients with *mild* disease (who have *not* received antibiotics in the previous 4 to 6 weeks) include: amoxicillin/clavulanate (1.75 to 4 g/250 mg/day), amoxicillin (1.5 to 4 g/day), cefpodoxime proxetil, cefuroxime axetil, or cefdinir. For patients with β-lactam allergies, trimethoprim/sulfamethoxazole (TMP/SMX), doxycycline, azithromycin, clarithromycin, or erythromycin may be considered, but bacteriologic failure rates of 20% to 25% are possible. Telithromycin is a new antibiotic that can also be used. Further PK/PD data is still required. Failure to respond to antimicrobial therapy after 72 hours should lead to either a switch to alternate antimicrobial therapy or the reevaluation of the patient. Initial therapy for adults with *mild* disease who *have* received antibiotics in the previous 4 to 6 weeks or adults with *moderate* disease includes the following choices: respiratory fluoroquinolone (eg, gatifloxacin, levofloxacin, moxifloxacin) or high-dose amoxicillin/clavulanate (4 g/250 mg/day).

Pharmacologic Therapy for Children

Initial therapy for children with *mild* disease who have *not* received antibiotics in the previous 4 to 6 weeks includes the following: high-dose amoxicillin/clavulanate (90 mg/6.4 mg/kg/day), amoxicillin (90 mg/kg/day), cefpodoxime proxetil, cefuroxime axetil,

FIGURE 12.1 — Sinus and Allergy Health Partnership*—Recommended Antibiotic Therapy for Adults With ABRS†

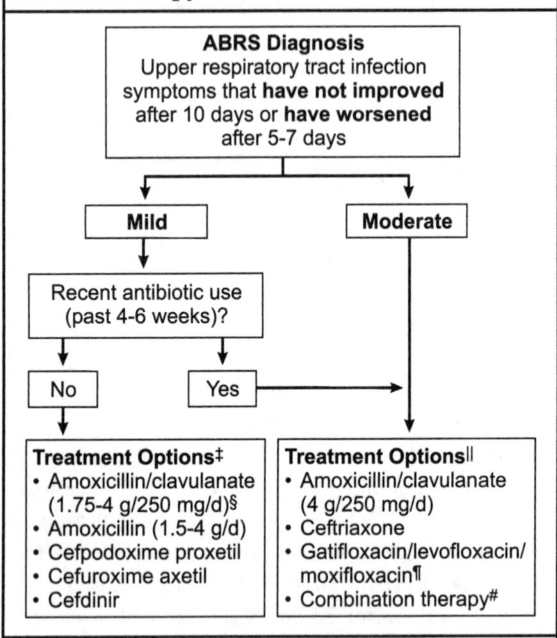

Abbreviation: ABRS, acute bacterial rhinosinusitis.

* The Sinus and Allergy Health Partnership, a conjoint group initially sponsored by the American Academy of Otolaryngology—Head and Neck Surgery, the American Academy of Otolaryngic Allergy, and the American Rhinologic Society, and individuals from the fields of infectious disease, pediatric infectious disease, microbiology, and pharmacy, have developed these guidelines as an educational tool for health care providers involved in managing patients with ABRS.

† This algorithm is based on the full guidelines published in *Otolaryngology—Head and Neck Surgery*. Readers should consult the full published guidelines for complete recommendations.

Continued

‡ In patients with mild disease, no recent exposure to antibiotics, and a history of β-lactam allergies, trimethoprim/sulfamethoxazole, doxycycline, a macrolide, or telithromycin are recommended.

§ Higher daily doses of amoxicillin (4 g/d) may be advantageous in areas with a high prevalence of penicillin-resistant *Streptococcus pneumoniae* or drug-resistant *S pneumoniae*, for patients with moderate disease, for patients who may need better *Haemophilus influenzae* coverage, or for patients with risk factors for infection with a resistant pathogen. There is a greater potential for treatment failure or resistant pathogens in these patient groups.

|| In patients with a history of β-lactam allergies and either mild disease with recent antibiotic exposure or moderate disease, fluoroquinolones or clindamycin plus rifampin are recommended.

¶ Concern has been raised about the potential for selecting quinolone resistance in patients treated with any quinolone for any reason within the past 4 to 6 weeks.

Based on *in vitro* spectrum of activity, combination therapy with appropriate coverage for gram-positive and gram-negative pathogens may be appropriate. Examples of combination-therapy regimens include high-dose amoxicillin (4 g/d) or clindamycin plus cefixime, or high-dose amoxicillin (4 g/d) or clindamycin plus rifampin. There is no clinical evidence at this time, however, of the safety or efficacy of these combinations.

Sinus and Allergy Health Partnership. *Otolaryngol Head Neck Surg*. 2004;130(suppl 1):1-45.

12

TABLE 12.2 — Recommended Antibiotic Therapy for Adults With ABRS

Initial Therapy	Calculated Clinical Efficacy (%)*	Calculated Bacteriologic Efficacy (%)*	Switch-Therapy Options (No Improvement or Worsening After 72 Hours)[†]
Mild disease[‡] with no recent antimicrobial use (past 4-6 weeks)[§]			
Amoxicillin/clavulanate (1.75-4 g/250 mg/d)[§‖]	90-91	97-99	Gatifloxacin, levofloxacin, moxifloxacin Amoxicillin/clavulanate 4 g/250 mg Ceftriaxone Combination therapy[¶]
Amoxicillin (1.5-4 g/d)[‖]	87-88	91-92	
Cefpodoxime proxetil	87	91	
Cefuroxime axetil	85	87	
Cefdinir	83	85	
β-Lactam allergic[#]			
TMP/SMX	83	84	Gatifloxacin, levofloxacin, moxifloxacin Rifampin plus clindamycin
Doxycycline	81	80	
Azithromycin, clarithromycin, erythromycin	77	73	
Telithromycin	See footnote.**	73	

Mild disease[‡] with recent antimicrobial use (past 4-6 weeks) or moderate disease[‡]			
Gatifloxacin, levofloxacin, moxifloxacin	92	100	Reevaluate patient[‡‡]
Amoxicillin/clavulanate (4 g/250 mg)	91	99	
Ceftriaxone	91	99	
(Combination therapy)[¶]	N/A	N/A	
β-Lactam allergic[#]			
Gatifloxacin, levofloxacin, moxifloxacin	92	100	Reevaluate patient[‡‡]
Clindamycin and rifampin[††]	N/A	N/A	

Abbreviations: ABRS, acute bacterial rhinosinusitis; CT, computed tomography; N/A, not available; TMP/SMX, trimethoprim/sulfamethoxazole.

* Clinical and bacterial efficacy (ie, clinical and microbiologic adequacy) is represented by the calculation from the Poole Therapeutic Outcome Model using the mean values of two surveillance data sets: the US component of the Alexander project (1998 to 2001) and SENTRY surveillance data. These values to not guarantee clinical success or failure. The Poole Therapeutic outcome model has been utilized as a recommended methodology in numerous academic guidelines. This model has not been clinically validated.

Continued

† When a change in antibiotic therapy is made, the clinician should consider the limitations in coverage of the initial antibiotic. The respiratory fluoroquinolones (gatifloxacin, levofloxacin, and moxifloxacin), ceftriaxone, and amoxicillin/clavulanate (4 g/250 mg) currently have the best coverage for both *Streptococcus pneumoniae* and *Haemophilus influenzae*. The terms mild and moderate are designed to aid in selecting antibiotic therapy.

‡ The difference in severity of disease does not imply the presence or absence of antimicrobial resistance. Rather, this terminology indicates the relative degree of acceptance of possible therapeutic failure and the likelihood of achieving spontaneous resolution of symptoms. The determination of disease severity lies with the clinician's evaluation of the patient's history and clinical presentation. Severe, life-threatening infection, with or without complications, is not addressed in these guidelines.

§ Prior antibiotic therapy within 4 to 6 weeks is a risk factor for infection with resistant organisms. Antibiotic choices should be based on this and other risk factors.

‖ The total daily dose of amoxicillin and the amoxicillin component of amoxicillin/clavulanate can vary from 1.5 to 4 g/day. Lower daily doses (1.5 g/day) are more appropriate in mild disease in patients with no risk factors for infection with a resistant pathogen (including recent antibiotic use). Higher daily doses (4 g/day) may be advantageous in areas with a high prevalence of penicillin-resistant *S pneumoniae* or drug-resistant *S pneumoniae*, for patients with moderate disease, for patients who may need better *H influenzae* coverage or for patients with risk factors for infection with a resistant pathogen. There is a greater potential for treatment failure or resistant pathogens in these patient groups.

¶ Based on *in vitro* spectrum of activity; combination therapy using appropriate gram-positive and gram-negative coverage may be appropriate. Examples of combination therapy regimens include high-dose amoxicillin (4 g/day) or clindamycin plus cefixime, or high-dose amoxicillin (4 g/day) or clindamycin, plus rifampin. There is no clinical evidence at this time, however, of the safety or efficacy of these combinations.

Cephalosporins should be considered initially for patients with penicillin intolerance/non-Type I hypersensitivity reactions (eg, rash). TMP/SMX, doxycycline, macrolides, azalides, and ketolides are not recommended unless the patient is β-lactam allergic. Their effectiveness against the major pathogens of ABRS is limited, and bacterial failure of 20% to 25% is possible. A respiratory fluoroquinolone (eg, gatifloxacin, levofloxacin, moxifloxacin) is recommended for patients who have allergies to β-lactams or who have recently failed other regimens.

** Further pharmacokinetic/pharmacodynamic data on this compound is needed.

†† Rifampin is a well-known inducer of several cytochrome P450 isoenzymes and therefore has a high potential for drug interactions.

‡‡ Reevaluation is necessary because the antibiotics recommended for initial therapy provide excellent activity against the predominant ABRS pathogens, including *S pneumoniae* or *H influenzae*. Additional history, physical examination, cultures, and/or CT scan may be indicated, and the possibility of other less common pathogens considered.

Sinus and Allergy Health Partnership. *Otolarangol Head Neck Surg*. 2004;130(suppl):S37.

TABLE 12.3 — Recommended Antibiotic Therapy for Children With ABRS

Initial Therapy	Calculated Clinical Efficacy (%)*	Calculated Bacteriologic Efficacy (%)*	Switch-Therapy Options (No Improvement or Worsening After 72 Hours)†
Mild disease‡ with no recent antimicrobial use (past 4-6 weeks)§			
Amoxicillin/clavulanate (90 mg/6.4 mg/kg/d)‖	91-92	97-99	Amoxicillin clavulanate (90 mg/6.4 mg/kg/d) Ceftriaxone Combination therapy¶
Amoxicillin‖	86-87	90-92	
Cefpodoxime proxetil	87	92	
Cefuroxime axetil	85	88	
Cefdinir	84	86	
β-Lactam allergic#			
TMP/SMX	83	84	Reevaluate patient** Combination therapy¶
Azithromycin, clarithromycin, erythromycin	78	76	

Mild disease[‡] with recent antimicrobial use (past 4-6 weeks) or moderate disease[‡]			
Amoxicillin/clavulanate (90 mg/6.4 mg/kg/d)[‖]	92	99	Reevaluate patient**
Ceftriaxone	91	99	
β-Lactam allergic[#]			
TMP/SMX	83	84	Reevaluate patient** Combination therapy[¶] (clindamycin or TMP/SMX plus rifampin)
Azithromycin, clarithromycin, erythromycin	78	76	
Clindamycin[††]	79	78	

Abbreviations: ABRS, acute bacterial rhinosinusitis; CT, computed tomography; TMP/SMX, trimethoprim/sulfamethoxazole.

* Clinical and bacterial efficacy (ie, clinical and microbiologic adequacy) is represented by the calculation from the Poole Therapeutic Outcome Model using the mean values of two surveillance data sets: the US component of the Alexander project (1998 to 2001) and SENTRY surveillance data. These values to not guarantee clinical success or failure.

† When a change in antibiotic therapy is made, the clinician should consider the limitations in coverage of the initial antibiotic. Ceftriaxone and high-dose amoxicillin/clavulanate currently have the best coverage for both *Streptococcal pneumoniae* and *Haemophilus influenzae*.

Continued

‡ The terms mild and moderate are designed to aid in selecting antibiotic therapy. The difference in severity of disease does not imply the presence or absence of antimicrobial resistance. Rather, this terminology indicates the relative degree of acceptance of possible therapeutic failure, and the likelihood of achieving spontaneous resolution of symptoms. The determination of disease severity lies with the clinician's evaluation of the patient's history and clinical presentation. Severe, life-threatening infection, with or without complications, is not addressed in these guidelines.

§ Prior antibiotic therapy within 4 to 6 weeks is a risk factor for infection with resistant organisms. Antibiotic choices should be based on this and other risk factors.

‖ The total daily dose of amoxicillin and the amoxicillin component of amoxicillin/clavulanate can vary from 45 to 90 mg/kg/day. Lower daily doses (45 mg/kg/day) are more appropriate in mild disease in patients with no risk factors for infection with a resistant pathogen (including recent antibiotic use). Higher daily doses (90 mg/kg/day) may be advantageous in areas with a high prevalence of penicillin-resistant *S pneumoniae* or drug resistant *S pneumoniae*, for patients with moderate disease, for patients who may need better *H influenzae* coverage or for patients with risk factors for infection with a resistant pathogen. There is a greater potential for treatment failure or resistant pathogens in these patient groups.

¶ Based on *in vitro* spectrum of activity; combination therapy using appropriate gram-positive and gram-negative coverage may be appropriate. Examples of combination therapy regimens include high-dose amoxicillin (90 mg/kg/day) or clindamycin plus cefixime, or high-dose amoxicillin (4 mg/kg/day) or clindamycin, plus rifampin. Other combination therapy regimens may be appropriate for patients with β-lactam allergy. There is no clinical evidence at this time, however, of the safety or efficacy of these combinations.

Cephalosporins should be considered initially for patients with penicillin intolerance/non-Type I hypersensitivity reactions (eg, rash). TMP/SMX, macrolides, and azalides are not recommended unless the patient is β-lactam allergic. Their effectiveness against the major pathogens of ABRS is limited, and bacterial failure of 20% to 25% is possible.

** Reevaluation is necessary because the antibiotics recommended for initial therapy provide excellent activity against the predominant ABRS pathogens, including *S pneumoniae* or *H influenzae*. Additional history, physical examination, cultures, and/or CT scan may be indicated, and the possibility of other less common pathogens considered.

†† Excluding β-lactams, clindamycin is the most active oral agent currently available with activity against approximately 90% of *S pneumoniae* isolates. It has no activity, however, against *H influenza*e or *M catarrhalis*.

Sinus and Allergy Health Partnership. *Otolarangol Head Neck Surg*. 2004;130(suppl):S37.

12

or cefdinir. The recommended initial therapy for children with *mild* disease who *have* received antibiotics in the previous 4 to 6 weeks *or* children with *moderate* disease is high-dose amoxicillin/clavulanate (90 mg/6.4 mg/kg/day). Cefpodoxime proxetil, cefuroxime axetil, or cefdinir may be considered initially for patients with penicillin intolerance/non–type 1 hypersensitivity reactions (eg, penicillin rash); in such instances, cefdinir is preferred because of high patient acceptance. TMP/SMX, azithromycin, clarithromycin, or erythromycin may be used if the patient is β-lactam allergic, but they do not provide optimal coverage.

Allergic Reactions to β-Lactam Antibiotics

Clinicians are concerned about potential allergic reactions to β-lactam antibiotics in the treatment of respiratory infections. These reactions range in the most part from the delayed typical morbilliform rash that may develop after several days of therapy to the more rare form of urticaria or angioedema characteristic of immediate type-1 hypersensitivity reaction mediated by IgE.

Guidelines for treatment of ABRS and acute otitis media specifically endorse the use of second- and third-generation cephalosporins. These β-lactam antimicrobials have a good safety record, yet many physicians are reluctant to prescribe cephalosporins in patients with a history of a rash to penicillin, depriving them of optimal antibiotic therapy.

Early studies of allergic reactions between the penicillins and cephalosporins suggested 8% to 10% risk of cross-reactivity, but most reactions were not type-1, and were probably related to the presence of penicillin contamination in the first-generation compounds. Later studies involving the second- and third-generation cephalosporins (cefdinir, cefpodoxime proxetil, cefuroxime axetil) demonstrate a very low rate of cross-reactivity (Weiss and Adkinson, 1998).

It is considered safe to prescribe a cephalosporin in a patient who has not had prior type-1 immediate reactions to these β-lactams, and it is suggested to query the patient regarding prior history of allergic reactions to antibiotics. Most nonimmune reactions can easily be treated with cessation of the antimicrobial.

Summary

It is the usual practice to treat for 7 to 10 days. Newer research shows that therapy for 5 days with an effective antibiotic is reasonable. Persistent symptoms are often likely due to persistent inflammation rather than to persistent infection.

12

13 Chronic Rhinosinusitis

Chronic rhinosinusitis (CRS) is an umbrella term for a number of pathologic conditions in which inflammation of the nose and paranasal sinuses is the final common pathway. These include:

- Allergy
- Immunodeficiency states
- Neoplasms
- Viruses
- Bacteria
- Fungi
- Genetic/congenital abnormalities
- Mucociliary dysfunction
- Noxious chemicals
- Pollutants
- Smoking.

Subgroups of these categories, such as superantigen formation, bacterial biofilms, and allergic fungal disease, have been identified.

The diagnosis of CRS has been defined by consensus in order to develop a framework of terminology that clinicians and researchers can utilize for standardized communication (**Table 13.1**). CRS is when symptoms have been present for 12 weeks and there is physical evidence (usually by nasal endoscopy) of mucosal swelling, nasal discharge, or polyps. Mucosal abnormalities of the middle meatus or bulla are also concrete signs of inflammatory disease. Generalized or localized edema, erythema, or granulation tissue can be caused by other rhinologic diseases, such as allergic rhinitis, and therefore requires imaging confirmation.

TABLE 13.1 — Measures for Diagnosing Chronic Rhinosinusitis for Adult Clinical Care

- Duration of disease is qualified by continuous symptoms for >12 consecutive weeks or >12 weeks of physical findings.*
- One of these signs of inflammation must be present and identified in association with ongoing symptoms consistent with CRS:
  - Discolored nasal drainage arising from the nasal passages, nasal polyps, or polypoid swelling as identified on physical examination with anterior rhinoscopy or nasal endoscopy. Anterior rhinoscopy should be performed in the decongested state.
  - Edema or erythema of the middle meatus or ethmoid bulla as identified by nasal endoscopy.
  - Generalized or localized erythema, edema, or granulation tissue. If it does not involve the middle meatus or ethmoid bulla, radiologic imaging is required to confirm a diagnosis.†
- Imaging modalities for confirming the diagnosis:
  - CT scan: demonstrating isolated or diffuse mucosal thickening, bone changes, air-fluid level.
  - Plain sinus radiograph: Water's view revealing mucous membrane thickening of >5 mm or complete opacification of one or more sinuses. An air-fluid level is more predictive of acute rhinosinusitis but may also be seen in CRS.‡
  - MRI is not recommended as an alterative to CT for routine diagnosis of CRS because of its excessively high sensitivity and lack of specificity.

Abbreviations: CRS, chronic rhinosinusitis; CT, computed tomography; MRI, magnetic resonance imaging.

* Signs consistent with CRS will support the symptom time duration

† Other chronic rhinologic conditions such as allergic rhinitis can result in such findings, and therefore they may not be associated with rhinosinusitis. It is recommended that a diagnosis of rhinosinusitis require radiologic confirmation under these circumstances

Continued

‡ A plain sinus radiograph without the equivocal signs listed here is not considered diagnostic. Aside from an air-fluid level, plain sinus radiographs have low sensitivity and specificity.

Benninger MS et al. *Otolaryngol Head Neck Surg*. 2003; 129:S5.

The best radiologic study for the evaluation of the sinuses is a computed tomography (CT) scan (**Figure 13.1**). Plain film sinus radiographs may be helpful in some instances for confirming the diagnosis of symptomatic patients with equivocal physical findings. Magnetic resonance imaging (MRI) scans may be too sensitive. Given the role of CT scanning in identifying mucosal abnormalities in the sinuses, MRI scans are not currently recommended.

A treatment paradigm for CRS is difficult, since there are numerous underlying etiologies. Since inflammation is present, anti-inflammatory therapy is key in the clinician's arsenal. Frequently, a "shot-gun" approach is undertaken. One regimen might include antibiotic therapy for 10 to 21 days, systemic steroids, leukotriene modifiers, nasal irrigations (such as saline with antifungals, antibacterials, or diuretics), and nasal steroids. Repeat evaluation of the patient with or without CT scan is performed a number of weeks after this "maximal" therapy.

Surgery is a last resort and is reserved for patients who have not responded to therapy. Obviously, neoplasms and certain other pathologies are absolute indications for surgical intervention. Surgery is usually performed via an minimally invasive endoscopic approach. The use of computer-aided surgical devices (manufactured by companies such as BrainLab, GE, Medtronic Xomed, and Stryker) has revolutionized the manner in which endoscopic surgery is performed.

FIGURE 13.1 — Computer-Aided Endoscopic Sinus Surgery

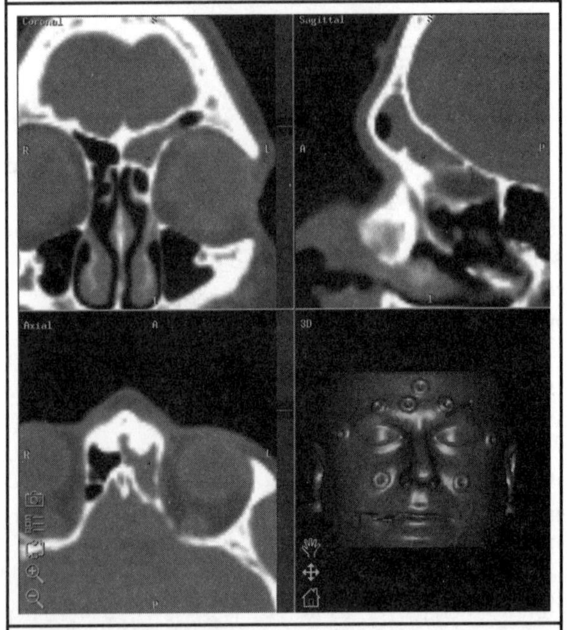

Courtesy of JB Anon, MD.

14 Case Studies

Case #1

A 47-year-old male, complaining of symptoms of facial pain, facial pressure, and nasal congestion with thickened discolored nasal secretions that have been persistent for the past 5 days, is seen for the fourth time within the past 5 months by his physician. Each of his previous episodes had improved after appropriate management with analgesics and topical nasal hydration with nasal saline; when his symptoms lasted >7 days, an antibiotic was administered.

The patient is in no acute distress, but presents with some significant nasal congestion, mouth breathing due to the congestion, and complaints of facial pain while bending forward.

Examination reveals markedly swollen nasal membranes, reddened posterior oropharynx, and tenderness on percussion of the maxillary sinuses.

Due to the persistence of his symptoms, the physician decides to send the patient for a computed tomography (CT) scan to determine the cause. The CT scan (**Color Plate 8**) demonstrates air-fluid levels in both maxillary sinuses, and very minimal-to-no ethmoid sinus disease.

Appropriate management of this patient's symptoms would be the use of topical nasal saline, oral decongestant therapy to reduce the congestive rhinitis, and possible adjunctive use of intranasal corticosteroids to help reduce the inflammatory component and reduce the potential for recurrence. Additionally, antimicrobial therapy would be based on the guidelines for treatment of acute bacterial rhinosinusitis (ABRS) based on the Sinus and Allergy Health Partnership data. Antibiotics directed against *Streptococcus pneumoniae* and *Haemophilus influenzae* for a total of 10 to 14 days would be appropriate in this patient.

This patient actually has had several acute viral respiratory tract infections with secondary complications of rhinosinusitis. He has no evidence of any significant obstructive disease and is not a candidate for consideration of surgical intervention. Very commonly, this type of patient has an episode during a "bad season." Usually, the symptoms regress over time with appropriate management.

Case # 2

A 23-year-old college student developed symptoms of acute upper respiratory tract congestion, facial discomfort, and thick discolored postnasal drainage and discharge. The symptoms persisted for 3 to 5 days and he sought the opinion of his physician. He was originally given erythromycin, which gave rise to significant stomach intolerance, and he discontinued this medication. As his symptoms persisted, he was then prescribed a cephalosporin antimicrobial that slowly improved symptoms. However, his nasal congestion, facial discomfort, symptoms of facial pressure, and discolored nasal discharge never went away. The patient has no prior history of significant symptoms of respiratory tract infections, he has no history of seasonal allergic rhinitis, nor is there a family history of allergic rhinitis.

Due to the persistence of symptoms of pain, facial pressure, and nasal discharge, he was seen by his family physician and referred for allergy evaluation, as well as a CT scan.

Allergy testing was found to be unremarkable: only minor reactivity to house-dust mites and molds. The CT scan (now 2 months after the onset of symptoms) demonstrated complete opacification of both ethmoid sinuses, partial opacification of both maxillary sinuses, and air-fluid levels and obstruction of both osteomeatal complexes (**Color Plate 9**).

The patient was referred to an otolaryngologist for further evaluation and discussion of possible surgical drainage. The examination revealed bilateral nasal congestion with marked hypertrophy of both inferior turbinates, and discolored, thick nasal drainage that was cultured (**Color Plate 10**).

This patient clearly has a diagnosis of chronic rhinosinusitis with both major and minor symptoms that have been present for >3 months.

Initial therapy included culture-directed antimicrobial therapy. A culture swab showed gram-negative clusters suggestive of *Moraxella catarrhalis*. Appropriate antibiotics directed against this organism were chosen. Additional therapy consisted of topical nasal lavage and irrigation with saline nasal rinses four times per day, topical decongestant therapy, and a short course of oral steroids. The patient required 14 days of antibiotic therapy and started to improve significantly. The ancillary medical therapy was continued for an additional 6 weeks with marked resolution of symptoms.

Case #3

A 13-year-old male developed nasal congestion, facial pressure described as headache, and a low-grade fever. He was thought to have a viral syndrome and was told to use analgesics and decongestant therapy. Three days later, he developed worsening of symptoms, marked left nasal obstruction, and thick discolored nasal discharge with persistent left facial pain in the maxillary region.

Despite treatment with amoxicillin, his symptoms continued. The patient was brought to the emergency department by his parents when they noted left eye swelling and partial closure on the fourth day of his symptoms (**Color Plate 11**). The boy had no previous symptoms of rhinosinusitis and had no prior history of allergic rhinitis.

In the emergency room, consultations were obtained with the ophthalmology department to rule out any orbital process (**Figure 14.1** and **Figure 14.2**).

The patient was diagnosed with ABRS with extension of infection into the left orbit. He was taken to the operating room immediately for drainage of the left maxillary and ethmoid sinuses and endoscopic drainage of a left periorbital subperiosteal abscess. Cultures obtained at surgery were positive for *S pneumoniae*, and he was subsequently started on high-dose penicillin therapy with excellent resolution of symptoms within 24 hours.

This patient demonstrates a complication of ABRS and development of orbital subperiorbital abscess. Compared with adults, children and adolescents pose an increased risk for bacterial infection to extend beyond the sinuses and to invade either the orbit (with formation of subperiosteal or orbital abscess) or brain (with development of intracranial empyema or abscess). Rapid recognition of signs and symptoms leads to appropriate referral and consultation with the specialty teams. Surgical therapy and drainage may be indicated in some of these cases. Appropriate management consists of intravenous hydration and antibiotics directed against the most common of the respiratory pathogens, topical nasal irrigation and lavage, as well as anti-inflammatory therapy.

Case #4

A 40-year-old white male presents to the clinic with the chief complaint of nasal symptoms. The patient states that he has had sneezing and itching of the

FIGURE 14.1 — Coronal Computed Tomography Scan Demonstrating Bilateral Maxillary Sinus Opacification

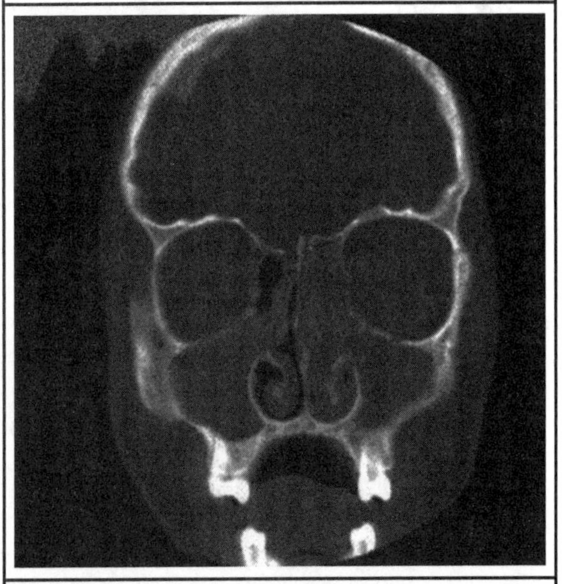

Coronal computed tomography (CT) scan demonstrates bilateral maxillary sinus opacification, left ethmoid sinus opacification, and infiltration into the left orbit.

Courtesy JA Hadley, MD.

nose and eyes for many years. He also has nasal congestion that causes him to mouth-breathe and snore at night. He will frequently wake up with a dry mouth. He feels that his nasal symptoms are present year round but may worsen with eye itching and tearing and clear rhinorrhea during the spring, summer, and fall months, particularly if he is outdoors. These symptoms are bothersome as the patient is an avid golfer and also mows his own lawn. He complains that he will have sneezing and increased nasal congestion during the winter months if he is vacuuming or cleaning his

FIGURE 14.2 — Axial Computed Tomography Scan Demonstrating Left Ophthalmopathy

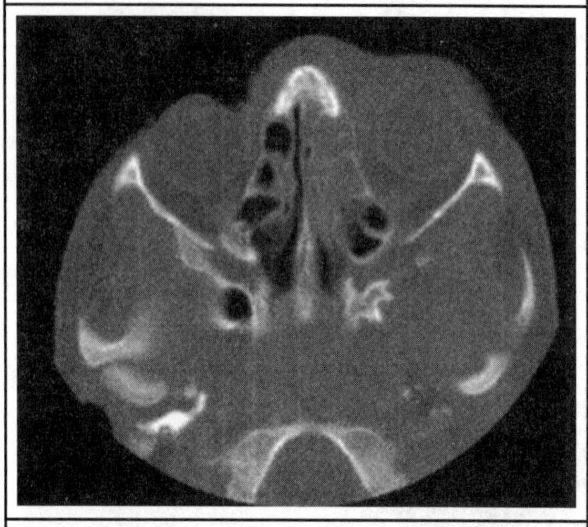

Axial computed tomography (CT) scan demonstrates left ophthalmopathy with opacified left ethmoid sinus and infiltration of infection into the left orbit.

Courtesy JA Hadley, MD.

home. The patient believes that cats also aggravate his nasal and eye symptoms; he will have immediate sneezing, itching, and sometimes wheezing upon entering his sister-in-law's home where there are two cats. He also notes that he may have some wheezing associated with cutting the grass.

The patient has tried over-the-counter remedies, such as Actifed and Tylenol Allergy Sinus. These medications help relieve some of his symptoms but also make him jittery and give him insomnia. Past medical and surgical history is remarkable for occasional increase in blood pressure and an appendectomy. There are no known drug allergies. The patient works as an insurance agent. He does not smoke and drinks alcohol only on the weekends. He is married and has two children <10 years of age.

Environmental history is significant for living in a century-old home, which, however, does have central heating and air-conditioning. There are no pets in his home. There is carpeting in the bedroom. On physical examination, the patient is in no acute distress. Blood pressure is 140/90 mm Hg. Head, eye, ear, nose, and throat examination is within normal limits except for boggy inferior turbinates that fill his anterior nasal cavity. Lungs are clear on exam. Skin is without rash, hives, or eczema. Remainder of his exam is normal.

Physician evaluation includes:

- Skin testing for common indoor and outdoor inhalant allergens, which include cat, dog, dust mite, mold, tree, grass, and weed allergens
- Laboratory tests: complete blood cell count with differential, complete metabolic panel (CMP), spirometry, and chest radiograph.

Assessment concludes that the patient has seasonal and perennial allergic rhinitis since his skin tests are positive for cat, mite, Alternaria, tree, grass, and weed allergens. Laboratory tests are all normal.

Mite and animal avoidance measures are reviewed. Medications are prescribed, including an oral antihistamine, a nasal steroid spray, and antihistamine eye drops. A leukotriene antagonist may be used if these medications do not provide enough symptomatic relief.

With the patient's history of wheezing, there should be consideration of a methacholine challenge test.

15 Resources

Allergy and Asthma Network/Mothers of Asthmatics, Inc. (AAN/MA)
3554 Chain Bridge Road, Suite 200
Fairfax, VA 22030
Phone: 800-878-4403 or 703/385-4403
Fax: 703/352-4354
Website: www.podi.com/health/aanma

A nonprofit organization founded in 1985 to help families in their quest to overcome and maintain control of asthma, allergies, and related conditions. AAN/MA produces *The MA Report*, a monthly newsletter for family education. A wide variety of books and videos are available from the learning resource center.

American Academy of Allergy, Asthma & Immunology (AAAAI)
611 East Wells Street
Milwaukee, WI 53202
Phone: 414/272-6071
Fax: 414/276-3349
Website: www.aaaai.org

Publishes *Asthma and Allergy ADVOCATE*; the toll-free number can be used for physician referral and information. The AAAAI offers brochures, booklets, newsletters, and videos; additional booklets are available for schools and nebulizer school nurses.

American Academy of Otolaryngic Allergy (AAOA)
1990 M Street, NW, Suite 680
Washington, DC 20036
Phone: 202/955-5010
Website: www.aaoaf.org

This is a major organization of ear, nose, and throat physicians dealing with allergic disorders pertaining to the field of otolaryngology. It is the oldest organized allergy society and has considerable information regarding the management of ear, nose, and throat allergic disorders and sino-nasal disease.

American Academy of Pediatrics (AAP)
141 North West Point Blvd.
Elk Grove Village, IL 60007
Phone: 847/228-5008
Fax: 847/228-7035
Website: www.aap.org

Brochures on asthma/allergy are available.

American Academy of Otolaryngology Head and Neck Surgery (AAOHNS)
One Prince Street.
Alexandria, VA 22314-3357
Phone: 703/836-4444
Website: www.entnet.org

This is a major resource for information concerning the disorders of the nose and paranasal sinuses. It is the largest organization for ear, nose, and throat physicians in the world and has a vast array of resources and information on line at the web address.

American College of Allergy and Immunology (ACAI)
85 West Algonquin Road, Suite 350
Arlington Heights, IL 60005
Phone: 847/427-1200 or 1-800-842-7777
Fax: 847/427-1294
Website: allergy.mcg.edu

Booklets and other materials on allergies and asthma; most information in booklets and other materials appears on the website. The toll-free number may be used for ordering booklets and materials on asthma and a list of allergists by state. ACAI provides educational materials and forms for use in schools. It also sponsors regional asthma education conferences for the public. The Website is maintained by allergists, the medical specialists who treat allergies and asthma, and their professional association, the American College of Allergy, Asthma and Immunology.

American Rhinologic Society (ARS)
Marvin P. Fried, MD, Secretary
Dept of Otolaryngology
Montefiore Medical Center
3400 Bainbridge Avenue
MAP 3rd Floor
Bronx, NY 10467-2490
Phone: 718/920-2991
Website: www.american-rhinologic.org

This Society is the largest professional organization dealing specifically with the nose. It is over 50 years old and the physician membership interests deal exclusively with rhinosinusitis, infection, and allergic disorders of the nose and paranasal sinuses. The website hosts reference material not only for clinicians, but also for lay persons and has links to other resources dealing with these disorders.

Asthma and Allergy Foundation of America (AAFA)
1125 15th Street NW, Suite 502
Washington, DC 20005
Phone: 202/466-7643 or 1-800-7-ASTHMA
Fax: 202/466-8940
Website: www.aafa.org

Resource for pamphlets, books, and other materials on asthma and allergies with special emphasis on material for children and teens; videos and educational interactive CD-ROM games for children available; resource list and prices available upon request; bimonthly newsletter with AAFA membership.

Sinus and Allergy Health Partnership (SAHP)
1990 M Street, NW, Suite 680
Washington, DC 20036
Phone: 202/955-5010
Fax: 202/955-5016
Website: www.sahp.org

The SAHP was formed in 1998 as an initiative by the AAOA, AAO-HNC, and ARS to provide awareness to both public and health care providers, enabling them to make educated decisions about treatment of allergies and sinus disease. Current treatment guidelines are posted on the website, as well as educational material of all types for the patient, primary care practitioner, and specialist.

16 References

Anticholinergics

Baroody F, Majchel A, Roecker M, et al. Ipratropium bromide (Atrovent® Nasal Spray) reduces the nasal response to methacholine. *J Allergy Clin Immunol.* 1992;89:1065-1075.

Baroody F, Ford S, Lichtenstein LM, et al. Physiologic responses and histamine release after nasal antigen challenge: effect of atropine. *Am J Respir Crit Care Med.* 1994;149: 1457-1465.

Bronsky EA, Druce H, Findlay SR, et al. A clinical trial of ipratropium bromide nasal spray in patients with perennial nonallergic rhinitis. *J Allergy Clin Immunol.* 1995;95: 1117-1122.

Grossman J, Banov C, Boggs P, et al. Use of ipratropium bromide nasal spray in chronic treatment of nonallergic perennial rhinitis, alone and in combination with other perennial rhinitis medications. *J Allergy Clin Immunol.* 1995; 95:1123-1127.

Meltzer EO, Orgel HA, Bronsky EA, et al. Ipratropium bromide aqueous nasal spray for patients with perennial allergic rhinitis: a study of its effect on their symptoms, quality of life, and nasal cytology. *J Allergy Clin Immunol.* 1992; 90:242-249.

Antihistamines

American Academy of Allergy, Asthma, and Immunology. Academy Position Statement: The Use of Antihistamines in Patients With Asthma. November, 2002.
http://www.aaaai.org/media/resources/academy_statements/position_statements/antihistamines_asthma.asp

Banov CH, Lieberman P. Efficacy of azelastine nasal spray in the treatment of vasomotor (perennial nonallergic) rhinitis. *Ann Allergy Asthma Immunol.* 2001;86:28-35.

Barnes CL, McKenzie CA, Webster KD, Poinsett-Holmes K. Cetirizine: a new nonsedating antihistamine. *Ann Pharmacother.* 1993;27:464-470.

Berger WE, White MV; Rhinitis Study Group. Efficacy of azelastine nasal spray in patients with an unsatisfactory response to loratadine. *Ann Allergy Asthma Immunol.* 2003;91:205-211.

Bronsky E, Boggs P, Findlay S, et al. Comparative efficacy and safety of a once-daily loratadine-pseudoephedrine combination versus its components alone and placebo in the management of seasonal allergic rhinitis. *J Allergy Clin Immunol.* 1995;96:139-147.

Busse WW. Role of antihistamines in allergic disease. *Ann Allergy.* 1994;72:371-375.

Ciprandi G, Pronzato C, Passalacqua G, et al. Topical azelastine reduces eosinophil activation and intercellar adhesion molecule-1 expression on nasal epithelial cells: an antiallergic activity [published erratum appears in *J Allergy Clin Immunol.* 1997;100:146]. *J Allergy Clin Immunol.* 1996;98(pt 1):1088-1096.

Ciprandi G, Ricca V, Passalacqua G, et al. Seasonal rhinitis and azelastine: long- or short-term treatment? *J Allergy Clin Immunol.* 1997;99:301-307

Fexofenadine. *The Medical Letter.* 1996;38:95.

Gastpar H, Nolte D, Aurich R, et al. Comparative efficacy of azelastine nasal spray and terfenadine in seasonal and perennial rhinitis. *Allergy.* 1994;49:152-158.

Holm AF, Fokkens WJ, Godthelp T, et al. A 1-year placebo-controlled study of intranasal fluticasone propionate aqueous nasal spray in patients with perennial allergic rhinitis: a safety and biopsy study. *Clin Otolaryngol.* 1998;23:69-73.

Honig PK, Wortham DC, Zamani K, et al. Terfenadine-ketoconazole interaction: pharmacokinetic and electrocardiographic consequences. *JAMA.* 1993;269:1513-1518.

LaForce CF, Corren J, Wheeler WJ, Berger WE; Rhinitis Study Group. Efficacy of azelastine nasal spray in seasonal allergic rhinitis patients who remain symptomatic after treatment with fexofenadine. *Ann Allergy Asthma Immunol.* 2004;93:154-159.

Larsen JS. Antihistamines: structural classification, pharmacokinetics and pharmacodynamics. *Hospital Medicine.* 1995;31(suppl):12-15.

Minshall E, Ghaffar O, Cameron L, et al. Assessment by nasal biopsy of long-term use of mometasone furoate aqueous nasal spray (Nasonex) in the treatment of perennial rhinitis. *Otolaryngol Head Neck Surg.* 1998;118:648-654.

Monahan BP, Ferguson CL, Killeary ES, et al. Torsades de pointes occurring in association with terfenadine use. *JAMA.* 1990;264:2788-2790.

Pelucchi A, Chiapparino A, Mastropasqua B, Marazzini L, Hernandez A, Foresi A. Effect of intranasal azelastine and beclomethasone dipropionate on nasal symptoms, nasal cytology, and bronchial responsiveness to methacholine in allergic rhinitis in response to grass pollens. *J Allergy Clin Immunol.* 1995;95:515-523.

Pipkorn U, Pukander J, Suonpaa J, et al. Long-term safety of budesonide nasal aerosol: a 5.5 year followup study. *Clin Allergy.* 1988;18:253-259.

Shin MH, Baroody F, Proud D, Kagey-Sobotka A, Lichtenstein LM, Naclerio RM. The effect of azelastine on the early allergic response. *Clin Exp Allergy.* 1992;22:289-295.

Simon FE, Simon KJ. The pharmacology and use of H_1-receptor antagonist drugs. *N Engl J Med.* 1994;330: 1663-1670.

Simons FER, McMillan JL, Simons KJ. A double-blind, single-dose, crossover comparison of cetirizine, terfenadine, loratadine, astemizole and chlorpheniramine versus placebo: suppressive effects on histamine-induced wheals and flares during 24 hours in normal subjects. *J Allergy Clin Immunol.* 1990;86:540-547.

Stern MA, Wade AG, Ridout SM, Cambell LM. Nasal budesonide offers superior symptom relief in perennial allergic rhinitis in comparison to nasal azelastine. *Ann Allergy Asthma Immunol.* 1998;81:354-358.

Tobin JR, Doyle TP, Ackerman AD, et al. Astemizole-induced cardiac conduction disturbances in a child. *JAMA.* 1991;226:2734-2740.

Wang D, Smitz J, De Waele M, Clement P. Effect of topical applications of budesonide and azelastine on nasal symptoms, eosinophil count and mediator release in atopic patients after nasal allergen challenge during the pollen season. *Int Arch Allergy Immunol.* 1997;114:185-192.

Weiner JM, Abramson MJ, Puy RM. Intranasal corticosteroids versus oral H1 receptor antagonists in allergic rhinitis: systematic review of randomised controlled trials. *BMJ.* 1998;317:1624-1629.

Woosley RL, Chen Y, Freiman JP, et al. Mechanism of the cardiotoxic actions of terfenadine. *JAMA.* 1993;269:1532-1536.

Antimicrobials

Alvarez-Elcoro S, Enzler MJ. The macrolides: erythromycin, clarithromycin, and azithromycin. *Mayo Clin Proc.* 1999;74:613-634.

American Academy of Pediatrics Subcommittee on Management of Acute Otitis Media. Clinical practice guideline: Diagnosis and management of acute otitis media. *Pediatrics.* 2004;113:1451-1466.

American Academy of Pediatrics Subcommittee on Management of Sinusitis and Comittee on Quality Improvement. Clinical practice guideline: Management of sinusitis. *Pediatrics.* 2001;108:798-808.

Doern GV, Brueggemann A, Holley HP, et al. Antimicrobial resistance of streptococcus pneumoniae recovered from outpatients in the United States during the winter months of 1994 to 1995: results of a 30-center National Surveillance Study. *Antimicrob Agents Chemother.* 1996;40:1208-1213.

File TM Jr, Segreti J, Dunbar L, et al. A multicenter, randomized study comparing the efficacy and safety of intravenous and/or oral levofloxacin versus ceftriaxone and/or cefuroxime axetil in treatment of adults with community-acquired pneumonia. *Antimicrob Agents Chemother.* 1997;41:1965-1972.

Goh YH, Goode RL. Current status of topical nasal antimicrobial agents. *Laryngoscope.* 2000;110:875-880.

Grepafloxacin—a new fluoroquinolone. *The Medical Letter.* 1998;40:17-18.

Gwaltney JM Jr, Scheld WM, Sande MA, Sydnor A. The microbial etiology and antimicrobial therapy of adults with acute community-acquired sinusitis: a fifteen-year experience at the University of Virginia and review of other selected studies. *J Allergy Clin lmmunol.* 1992;90:457-462.

Sinus and Allergy Health Partnership. Antimicrobial treatment guidelines for acute bacterial rhinosinusitis. Sinus and Allergy Health Partnership: Executive Summary. *Otolaryngol Head Neck Surg.* 2000;123(suppl):5-31.

Trovafloxin. *The Medical Letter.* 1998;40:30-31.

Walker RC. The fluoroquinolones. *Mayo Clin Proc.* 1999;74:1030-1037.

Weiss ME, Adkinson NF. Immediate hypersensitivity reactions to penicillin and related antibiotics. *Clin Allergy.* 1998;18:515-550.

Avoidance

Morgan WJ, Crain EF, Gruchalla RS, et al; Inner-City Asthma Study Group. Results of a home-based environmental intervention among urban children with asthma. *N Engl J Med.* 2004;351:1068-1080.

Platts-Mills TA. Allergen avoidance at home: what really works. *J Respir Dis.* 1989;10:53-55.

Platts-Mills TAE, Mitchell EB, Chapman MD, Heymann PW. Dust mite allergy: its clinical significance. *Hosp Pract.* 1987;22:91-100.

Sheikh A, Hurwitz B. House dust mite avoidance measures for perennial allergic rhinitis. Cochrane Database Syst Rev. 2001; CD001563.

Solomon WR, Bruge HA, Boise JR. Exclusion of particulate allergens by window air conditioners. *J Allergy Clin Immunol.* 1980;65:305-308.

Terreehorst I, Hak E, Oosting AJ, et al. Evaluation of impermeable covers for bedding in patients with allergic rhinitis. *N Engl J Med.* 2003;349:237-246.

Coexistent Rhinitis and Asthma

Bousquet J, Boushey HA, Busse WW, et al. Characteristics of patients with seasonal allergic rhinitis and concomitant asthma. *Clin Exp Allergy.* 2004;34:897-903.

Bousquet J, Van Cauwenberge P, Khaltaev N; Aria Workshop Group; World Health Organization. Allergic rhinitis and its impact on asthma. *J Allergy Clin Immunol.* 2001;108 (suppl 5):S147-S334.

Casale TB; Prous Science. Omalizumab: an effective anti-IgE treatment for allergic asthma and rhinitis. *Drugs Today (Barc).* 2004;40:367-376.

Greenberger PA. Interactions between rhinitis and asthma. *Allergy Asthma Proc.* 2004;25:89-93.

Huurre TM, Aro HM, Jaakkola JJ. Incidence and prevalence of asthma and allergic rhinitis: a cohort study of Finnish adolescents. *J Asthma.* 2004;41:311-317.

McCusker CT. Use of mouse models of allergic rhinitis to study the upper and lower airway link. *Curr Opin Allergy Clin Immunol.* 2004;4:11-16.

Passalacqua G, Ciprandi G, Pasquali M, Guerra L, Canonica GW. An update on the asthma-rhinitis link. *Curr Opin Allergy Clin Immunol.* 2004;4:177-183.

Vignola AM, Humbert M, Bousquet J, et al. Efficacy and tolerability of anti-immunoglobulin E therapy with omalizumab in patients with concomitant allergic asthma and persistent allergic rhinitis: SOLAR. *Allergy.* 2004;59:709-717.

Decongestants

Bronsky E, Boggs P, Findlay S, et al. Comparative efficacy and safety of a once-daily loratadine-pseudoephedrine combination versus its components alone and placebo in the management of seasonal allergic rhinitis. *J Allergy Clin Immunol.* 1995;96:139-147.

Hamilton LH, Chobanian SL, Cato A, et al. A study of sustained action pseudoephedrine in allergic rhinitis. *Ann Allergy*. 1982;48:87-92.

Kernan WN, Viscoli CM, Brass LM, et al. Phenylpropanolamine and the risk of hemorrhagic stroke. *N Engl J Med.* 2000;343:1826-1832.

Pentel P. Toxicity of over-the-counter stimulants. *JAMA*. 1984;252:1898-1903.

General Rhinitis

Chen H, Katz PP, Eisner MD, Yelin EH, Blanc PD. Health-related quality of life in adult rhinitis: The role of perceived control of disease. *J Allergy Clin Immunol*. 2004;114:845-850.

Druce HM, Hanifin JM, Meltzer EO, et al. Histamine-induced disease: impact of new research on treatment algorithms. *J Respir Dis*. 1992;13(suppl):S1-S39.

Dykewicz MS, Fineman S. Executive Summary of Joint Task Force Practice Parameters on Diagnosis and Management of Rhinitis. *Ann Allergy Asthma Immunol*. 1998;81:463-468.

Dykewicz MS, Fineman S, Skoner DP. Joint task force summary statements on diagnosis and management of rhinitis. *Ann Allergy Asthma Immunol*. 1998;81:474-518.

Garay R. Mechanisms of vasomotor rhinitis. *Allergy*. 2004;59(suppl 76):4-9; discussion 9-10.

Gendo K, Larson EB. Evidence-based diagnostic strategies for evaluating suspected allergic rhinitis. *Ann Intern Med*. 2004;140:278-289.

Johansson SG, Bieber T, Dahl R, et al. Revised nomenclature for allergy for global use: Report of the Nomenclature Review Committee of the World Allergy Organization, October 2003. *J Allergy Clin Immunol*. 2004;113:832-836.

Kaliner M, Lemanske R. Rhinitis and asthma. *JAMA*. 1992; 268:2807-2829.

Lombardi C. Relationship between kind and number of allergen positivity and bronchial responsiveness to methacholine in asthmatic or asthmatic plus rhinitis atopic patients. *Chest.* 1996;110:28S. Abstract.

Mathews KP. Respiratory atopic disease. *JAMA.* 1982; 248:2587-2610.

Meltzer EO. An overview of current pharmacotherapy in perennial rhinitis. *J Allergy Clin Immunol.* 1995;95:1097-1110.

Meltzer EO, Szwarcberg J, Pill MW. Allergic rhinitis, asthma, and rhinosinusitis: diseases of the integrated airway. *J Manag Care Pharm.* 2004;10:310-317.

Naclerio RM. Allergic rhinitis. *N Engl J Med.* 1991; 325:860-869.

Nathan RA, Meltzer EO, Selner JC, Storms W. Prevalence of allergic rhinitis in the United States. *J Allergy Clin Immunol.* 1997;99:S808-S814.

National Asthma Education Program: expert panel report. *Guidelines for the Diagnosis and Management of Asthma.* Bethesda, MD: National Institutes of Health; 1991:66.

Nelson HS. Diagnostic procedures in allergy. *Ann Allergy.* 1983;51:411-416.

Norman PS. Allergic rhinitis. *J Allergy Clin Immunol.* 1985; 75:531-545.

Rachelefsky GS. Pharmacologic management of allergic rhinitis. *J Allergy Clin Immunol.* 1998;101:S367-S369.

Slavin RG. Occupational and allergic impact on worker productivity and safety. *Allergy and Asthma Proc.* 1998;19:277-284.

Spector SL, Nicklas RA, Chapman JA, et al; Joint Task Force on Practice Parameters; American Academy of Allergy, Asthma, and Immunology; American College of Allergy, Asthma, and Immunology; Joint Council of Allergy, Asthma, and Immunology. Symptom severity assessment of allergic rhinitis: part 1. *Ann Allergy Asthma Immunol.* 2003;91:105-114.

Ten RM, Klein JS, Frigas E. Allergy skin testing. *Mayo Clin Proc.* 1995;70:783-784.

Van Arsdel PP, Larson EB. Diagnostic tests for patients with suspected allergic disease. *Ann Intern Med.* 1989;110: 304-312.

White MV, Kaliner MA. Mediators of allergic rhinitis. *J Allergy Clin Immunol.* 1992;90:699-704.

Young MC. Rhinitis, sinusitis and polyposis. *Allergy and Asthma Proc.* 1998;19:211-218

Histamine-1 Medications

Bousquet J, Bindslev-Jensen C, Canonica GW, et al. The ARIA/EAACI criteria for antihistamines: an assessment of the efficacy, safety and pharmacology of desloratadine. *Allergy.* 2004;59(suppl 77):4-16.

Day JH, Briscoe MP, Clark RH, et al. Onset of action and efficacy of terfenadine, astemizole, cetirizine, and loratadine for the relief of symptoms of allergic rhinitis. *Ann Allergy Asthma Immunol.* 1997;79:163-172.

Day JH, Briscoe MP, Widlitz MD. Cetirizine, loratadine or placebo in subjects with seasonal allergic rhinitis: effects after controlled ragweed pollen challenge in an environmental exposure unit. *J Allergy Clin Immunol.* 1998;101:638-645.

Druce HM, Thoden WR, Mure P, et al. Brompheniramine, loratadine and placebo in allergic rhinitis: a placebo-controlled comparative clinical trial. *Clin Pharmacology.* 1998;38:382-389.

Howarth PH, Stern MA, Roi L, et al. Double-blind, placebo-controlled study comparing the efficacy and safety of fexofenadine hydrochloride (120 and 180 mg once daily) and cetirizine in seasonal allergic rhinitis. *J Allergy Clin Immunol.* 1999;104:927-933.

Kaiser H, Harris AG, Capano D, et al. A double-blind placebo-controlled comparison of the safety and efficacy of loradtadine (Claritin), fexofenadine HCL (Allegra) and palcebo in the treatment of subjects with seasonal allergic rhinitis (SAR). *Allergy.* 1999;54(suppl 52):155. Abstract.

Klein GL, Littlejohn T 3rd, Lockhart EA, Furey SA. Brompheniramine, terfenadine and placebo in allergic rhinitis. *Ann Allergy Asthma Immunol.* 1996;77:337-340.

Persi L, Demoly P, Harris AG, et al. Comparison between nasal provocation tests and skin tests in patients treated with loratadine and cetirizine. *J Allergy Clin Immunol.* 1999;103: 591-594.

Prenner B, Capano D, Harris AG, et al. The safety and efficacy of loratadine (Claritin) versus fexofenadine (Allegra) in the treatment of seasonal allergic rhinitis (SAR): a multicenter crossover comparison with treatment of nonresponders. *Allergy.* 1999;54(suppl 52):295. Abstract.

Simon FE, McMillan JL, Simons KJ. A double-blind single-dose crossover comparison of cetirizine, terfenadine, loratadine, astemizole and chlorpheniramine versus placebo: suppressive effects on histamine-induced wheals and flares during 24 hours in normal subjects. *J Allergy Clin Immunol.* 1990;86:540-547.

Van Cauwenberge P, Juniper EF. Comparison of efficacy, safety and quality of life provided by fexofenadine hydrochloride 120 mg, loratadine 10 mg, and placebo administered once daily for the treatment of seasonal allergic rhinitis. *Clin Exp Allergy.* 2000;30:891-899.

Immunotherapy

Bousquet J, Lockey R, Hans-Jorgen M, WHO panel members. Allergen immunotherapy: therapeutic vaccines for allergic diseases. A WHO position paper. *J Allergy Clin Immunol.* 1998;102:558-562.

Fortner BR, Dantzler BS, Tipton WR, et al. The effect of weekly versus monthly ragweed allergen injections on immunological parameters. *Ann Allergy.* 1981;47:147-150.

Greenberg MA, Kaufman CR, Gonzalez GE, et al. Late and immediate systemic-allergic reactions to inhalant allergen immunotherapy. *J Allergy Clin Immunol.* 1986;77:865-870.

Metzger WJ, Turner E, Patterson R. The safety of immunotherapy during pregnancy. *J Allergy Clin Immunol.* 1978; 61:268-272.

Nelson HS. Diagnostic procedures in allergy: I. allergy skin testing. *Ann Allergy*. 1983;51:411-416.

Norman PS. Immunotherapy: past and present. *J Allergy Clin Immunol*. 1998;102:1-10.

Norman PS. Immunotherapy for nasal allergy. *J Allergy Clin Immunol*. 1988;81:992-996.

Leukotrienes

Nathan RA. Pharmacotherapy for allergic rhinitis: a critical review of leukotriene receptor antagonists compared with other treatments. *Ann Allergy Asthma Immunol*. 2003; 90:182-190.

Wilson AM, O'Byrne PM, Parameswaran K. Leukotriene receptor antagonists for allergic rhinitis: a systematic review and meta-analysis. *Am J Med*. 2004;116:338-344.

Nasal Corticosteroids

Andersson M, Berglund J, Greiff L, et al. A comparison of budesonide nasal dry powder with fluticasone propionate aqueous nasal spray in patients with perennial allergic rhinitis. *Rhinology*. 1995;33:18-21.

Day J, Carrillo T. Comparison of the efficacy of budesonide and fluticasone propionate aqueous nasal spray for once daily treatment of perennial allergic rhinitis. *J Allergy Clin Immunol*. 1998;102:902-908.

Drouin M, Yang WH, Bertrand B, et al. Once daily mometasone furoate aqueous nasal spray is as effective as twice daily beclomethasone dipropionate for treating perennial allergic rhinitis patients. *Ann Allergy Asthma Immunol*. 1996;77:153-160.

Dykewicz MS, Kaiser HB, Nathan RA, et al. Fluticasone propionate aqueous nasal spray improves nasal symptoms of seasonal allergic rhinitis when used as needed (prn). *Ann Allergy Asthma Immunol*. 2003;91:44-48.

Fluticasone propionate nasal spray for allergic rhinitis. *Medical Letter*. 1995;37:5-6.

Intranasal budesonide for allergic rhinitis. *Medical Letter*. 1994;36:63-64.

Jen A, Baroody F, de Tineo M, et al. As-needed use of fluticasone propionate nasal spray reduces symptoms of seasonal allergic rhinitis. *J Allergy Clin Immunol.* 2000;105: 732-738.

Juniper EF, Guyatt GH, Archer B, et al. Aqueous beclomethasone dipropionate in the tratment of ragweed pollen-induced rhinitis: further exploration of "as needed" use. *J Allergy Clin Immunol.* 1993;92:66-72.

Juniper EF, Kline PA, Hargreave FE, et al. Comparison of beclomethasone dipropionate aqueous nasal spray, astemizole, and the combination in the prophylactic treatment of ragweed pollen-induced rhinoconjunctivitis. *J Allergy Clin Immunol.* 1989;83:627-633.

Knight A, Kolin A. Long-term efficacy and safety of beclomethasone dipropionate aerosol in perennial rhinitis. *Ann Allergy.* 1983;50:81-84.

Mandl M, Nolop K, Lutsky B. Comparison of once daily mometasone furoate (Nasonex) and fluticasone propionate aqueous nasal sprays for the treatment of perennial rhinitis. *Ann Allergy Asthma Immunol.* 1997;79:370-378.

Nielsen LP, Dahl R. Comparison of intranasal corticosteroids and antihistamines in allergic rhinitis: a review of randomized, controlled trials. *Am J Respir Med.* 2003;2:55-65.

Norman PS, Winkenwerder WL, Agbayani BF, et al. Adrenal function during the use of dexamethasone aerosols in the treatment of ragweed hay fever. *J Allergy.* 1967;40:67-61.

Ratner PH, Paull BR, Findlay SR, et al. Fluticasone propionate given once daily is as effective for seasonal allergic rhinitis as beclomethasone dipropionate given twice daily. *J Allergy Clin Immunol.* 1992;90:285-291.

Scadding G, Lund V, Jacques L, et al. A placebo-controlled study of fluticasone propionate aqueous nasal spray and beclomethasone dipropionate in perennial rhinitis: efficacy in allergic and nonallergic perennial rhinitis. *Clin Exp Allergy.* 1995;25:737-743.

Sheth KK, Cook CK, Philpot EE, et al. Concurrent use of intranasal and orally inhaled fluticasone propionate does not affect hypothalamic-pituitary-adrenal-axis function. *Allergy Asthma Proc.* 2004;25:115-120.

Siegel SC. Topical intranasal corticosteroid therapy in rhinitis. *J Allergy Cin Immunol.* 1988;81:984-991.

Simpson RJ. Budesonide and terfenadine, separately and in combination, in the treatment of hay fever. *Ann Allergy.* 1994;73:497-502.

Stern MA, Dahl R, Nielsen LP, et al. A comparison of aqueous suspensions of budesonide spray (128 micrograms and 256 micrograms once daily) and fluticasone propionate nasal spray (200 micrograms once daily). *Am J Rhinology.* 1997;11:323-330.

Storms W, Bronsky E, Findlay S, et al. Once dainide nasal spray is effective for the treatment of perennial allergic rhinitis. *Ann Allergy.* 1991;66:329-334.

van Bavel J, Findlay SR, Hampel FC, et al. Intranasal fluticasone propionate is more effective than terfenadine tablets for seasonal allergic rhinitis. *Arch Intern Med.* 1994;154:2699-2704.

Waddell AN, Patel SK, Toma AG, Maw AR. Intranasal steroid sprays in the treatment of rhinitis: is one better than another? *J Laryngol Otol.* 2003;117:843-845.

Welsh PW, Stricker WE, Chu CP, et al. Efficacy of beclomethsone nasal solution, flunisolide and cromolyn in relieving symptoms of ragweed allergy. *Mayo Clin Proc.* 1987;62:125-134.

Wilson AM, Sims EJ, McFarlane LC, Lipworth BJ. Effects of intranasal corticosteroids on adrenal, bone, and blood markers of systemic activity in allergic rhinitis. *J Allergy Clin Immunol.* 1998;102:598-604.

Yanez A, Rodrigo GJ. Intranasal corticosteroids versus topical H1 receptor antagonists for the treatment of allergic rhinitis: a systematic review with meta-analysis. *Ann Allergy Asthma Immunol.* 2002;89:479-484.

Ocular Therapy

Bahmer FA, Ruprecht KW. Safety and efficacy of oral terfenadine. *Ann Allergy*. 1994;72:429-434.

Cromolyn sodium for allergic conjunctivitis. *Medical Letter*. 1985;27:7-8.

Ketorolac for seasonal allergic conjunctivitis. *Medical Letter*. 1993;35:88-89

Olopatadine for Allergic Conjunctivitis. *The Medical Letter.* 1997;39:108-109.

Ophthalmic levocabastine for allergic conjunctivitis. *Medical Letter*. 1994;36:35-36.

Omalizumab

Adelroth E, Rak S, Haahtela T, et al. Recombinant humanized mAb-E25, an anti-IgE mAb, in birch pollen-induced seasonal allergic rhinitis. *J Allergy Clin Immunol*. 2000;106: 253-259.

Casale TB, Condemi J, LaForce C, et al; Omalizumab Seasonal Allergic Rhinitis Trail Group. Effect of omalizumab on symptoms of seasonal allergic rhinitis: a randomized controlled trial. *JAMA*. 2001;286:2956-2967.

Casale TB, Bernstein IL, Busse WW, et al. Use of an anti-IgE humanized monoclonal antibody in ragweed-induced allergic rhinitis. J Allergy Clin Immunol. 1997;100:110-121.

Chervinsky P, Casale T, Townley R, et al. Omalizumab, an anti-IgE antibody, in the treatment of adults and adolescents with perennial allergic rhinitis. *Ann Allergy Asthma Immunol.* 2003;91:160-167.

Kuehr J, Brauburger J, Zielen S, et al. Efficacy of combination treatment with anti-IgE plus specific immunotherapy in polysensitized children and adolescents with seasonal allergic rhinitis. *J Allergy Clin Immunol.* 2002;109:274-280.

Kopp MV, Mayatepek E, Engels E, et al. Urinary leukotriene E4 levels in children with allergic rhinitis treated with specific immunotherapy and anti-IgE (Omalizumab). *Pediatr Allergy Immunol.* 2003;14:401-404.

Rhinosinusitis and Nasal Polyps

AHCPR. Diagnosis and treatment of acute bacterial rhinosinusitis. Rookville (MD): Agency for Health Care Policy and Research; 1999.

Ambrose PG, Anon JB, Owen JS, et al. Use of pharmacodynamic end points in the evaluation of gatifloxacin for the treatment of acute maxillary sinusitis. *Clin Infect Dis*. 2004;38:1513-1520.

Benninger MS, Ferguson BJ, Hadley JA, et al. Adult chronic rhinosinusitis: definitions, diagnosis, epidemiology, and pathophysiology. *Otolaryngol Head Neck Surg*. 2003;129 (suppl 3):S1-S32.

Brook I, Frazier EH, Foot PA. Microbiology of chronic maxillary sinusitis: comparison between specimens obtained by sinus endoscopy and by surgical drainage. *J Med Microbiol*. 1997;46:430-432.

Gwaltney JM Jr, Phillips CD, Miller RD, Riker DK. Computed tomographic study of the common cold. *N Engl J Med*. 1994;330:25-30.

Hoover GE, Newman LJ, Platts-Mills TAE, Phillips CD, Gross CW, Wheatley LM. Chronic sinusitis: risk factors for extensive disease. *J Allergy Clin Immunol*. 1997;100:185-191.

Jacobs MR, Anon J, Appelbaum PC. Mechanisms of resistance among respiratory tract pathogens. *Clin Lab Med*. 2004;24:419-453.

Kennedy DW. Functional endoscopic sinus surgery techniques. *Arch Otolaryngol*. 1985;111:643-649.

Lanza DC, Kennedy DW. Adult rhinosinusitis defined. *Otolaryngol Head Neck Surg*. 1997;117:S1-S7.

Lildholdt T, Fogstrup J, Gammelgaard N, et al. Surgical versus medical treatment of nasal polyps. *Acta Otolaryngol*. 1988;105:140-143.

Parameters for the diagnosis and management of sinusitis. *J Allergy Clin lmmunol*. 1998;102:S107-S144.

Ponikau JU, Sherris DA, Kern EB, et al. The diagnosis and incidence of allergic fungal sinusitis. *Mayo Clin Proc.* 1999;74:877-884.

Rachelefsky GS, Katz RM, Siegel SC. Chronic sinus disease with associated reactive airway disease in children. *Pediatrics.* 1984;73:526-529.

Ray NF, Baraniuk JN, Thamer M, et al. Healthcare expenditures for sinusitis in 1996: contribution of asthma, rhinitis, and other airway disorders. *J Allergy Clin Immunol.* 1999;103:408-414.

Settipane GA, Chafee FH. Nasal polyps in asthma and rhinitis: a review of 6,037 patients. *J Allergy Clin Immunol.* 1977;59:1721.

Shoseyov D, Bibi H, Shai P, Shoseyov N, Shazberg G, Hurvitz H. Treatment with hypertonic saline versus normal saline wash of pediatric chronic sinusitis. *J Allergy Clin Immunol.* 1998;101:602-605.

Sinus and Allergy Partnership. Antimicrobial treatment guidelines for acute bacterial rhinosinusitis. *Otolaryngol Head Neck Surg.* 2004;130(suppl 1):1-45.

Slavin RG. Recalcitrant asthma: could sinusitis be the culprit? *J Respir Dis.* 1991;12:182-194.

Slavin RG. Relationship of nasal disease and sinusitis to bronchial asthma. *Ann Allergy.* 1982;49:76-80.

Stewart MG, Donovan DT, Parke RB Jr, Bautista MH. Does the severity of sinus computed tomography findings predict outcome in chronic sinusitis? *Otolaryngol Head Neck Surg.* 2000;123:81-84

Tamooka LT, Murphy C, Davidson TM. Clinical study and literature review of nasal irrigation. *Laryngoscope.* 2000;110: 1189-1193.

Vogan JO, Bolger WE, Keyes AS. Endoscopically guided sinonasal cultures: a direct comparison with maxillary sinus aspirate cultures. *Otolaryngol Head Neck Surg.* 2000; 122:370-373.

Wald ER. Microbiology of acute and chronic sinusitis in children. *J Allergy Clin Immunol.* 1992;90:452-456.

Wagner W. Changing diagnostic and treatment strategies for chronic sinusitis. *Cleve Clinic J Med.* 1996;63:396-405.

Williams JW Jr, Simel DL, Roberts L, Samsa GP. Clinical evaluation for sinusitis. Making the diagnosis by history and physical examination. *Ann Intern Med.* 1992;117:705-710.

Zinreich SJ. Imaging of chronic sinusitis in adults: x-ray, computed tomography, and magnetic resonance imaging. *J Allergy Clin Immunol.* 1992;90:445-451.

INDEX

Note: Page numbers in *italics* indicate figures.
Page numbers followed by t refer to tables.
Numbers preceded by CP indicate Color Plates.

ABRS. See *Bacterial rhinosinusitis, acute.*
Acaricides, 40t, 41
Actifed, 144
Acular (ketorolac tromethamine), 74, 75t
Adenoid hypertrophy
  age and, 13, 27
  detection of, 32
Adolescents, adenoid hypertrophy in, 13, 27
Afrin. See *Oxymetazoline nasal spray.*
Age. See also *Adolescents; Children.*
  allergic rhinitis and, 15t, 16, 28-29
  chronic rhinitis syndromes and, 15t
  gustatory rhinitis and, 18
  nasal polyps and, 18
  otitis media and, 37
Air cell, in turbinate, 13
Air conditioning, 40
Air filters, in dust mite avoidance, 41
Air-fluid levels, in sinuses, CP4, CP7, CP8, CP9, *110,* 139, 141
Alamast (pemirolast potassium), 75t
Albuterol
  for asthma, 52
  in pregnancy, 76t-77t
Alcohol ingestion, 31
Alkylamines. See also specific drugs.
  dosages of, 46t
Allegra. See *Fexofenadine.*
Allergens
  animals as, 25t, 28-30, 34, 40, 80
  cockroaches as, 25t
  dust mites as, 25t, 30-31, 34, 40, 40t, 80
  food as, 31, 34
  geographic variations in, 30
  grass as, 25t, 30, 80
  medications as, 31
  mold as
    indoors, 25t
    outdoors, 25t, 31, 40
    seasonal, 25t, 31
    skin tests for, 34
    spore count in, 25t, 31
  perennial, 92t
  pollen as, 25t, 28t, 30, 34, 40, 80, 92t
  ragweed as, 16, 25t, 35, 53-54, 67, 80
  seasonal, 25t, 28t, 30-31, 92t
  trees as, 25t, 30, 80

Allergic conjunctivitis
in children, 74
environmental control measures and, 42
Allergic reactions. See also *Inflammatory cascade.*
components of, 21
early- and late-phase, *24,* 26
Allergic rhinitis, 92t
age and, 15t, 16, 28-29
antihistamines in, 50-54
causes of, 15t, 32-33. See also *Allergens.*
chronic, 135. See also *Rhinosinusitis, chronic.*
decongestants for, 57, 60
diagnosis of, 11
skin tests in. See *Allergy skin tests.*
differential diagnosis of, 28t
familial, 29
guidelines for, 37-38
incidence of, 11, 16, 29
inflammatory cascade in, 21-22, *22-24,* 24-26
inhalant sensitivities in, 16, 21
nasal discharge in, 33
seasonal
asthma with, 87
in children, 72
cromolyn sodium for, 70
desloratadine for, 51-52
fluticasone nasal spray for, 63
intranasal steroids for, 67-68
intranasal vs oral antihistamines for, 54-55
methacholine provocation in, 86
montelukast for, 72
omalizumab for, 88
symptoms of, 14t, 28-29, 142-144
treatment of. See *Rhinitis treatment.*
Allergic Rhinitis and Its Impact on Asthma (ARIA), 38, 68
Allergy and Asthma Network/Mothers of Asthmatics, Inc. (AAN/MA), 147
Allergy skin tests
advantages of, 33-35
discontinuing medications before, 33-34
in gustatory rhinitis, 18
indications for, 145
interpreting results of, 34
materials for, 34
nasal polyps and, 19
prick vs intradermal, 35
procedures in, 34-35
in rhinitis diagnosis, 11, 14t, 33-35
treatment decisions from, 39-40
units of measure in, 35
Allergy units (AU), 35
Alocril (nedocromil sodium), 75t-77t
Alrex (lotepredol), 75t

Alternaria, 25t, 31, 145
American Academy of Allergy, Asthma, and Immunology (AAAAI), 37, 147
American Academy of Otolaryngic Allergy (AAOA), 147
American Academy of Otolaryngology Head and Neck Surgery (AAOHNS), 148
American Academy of Pediatrics (AAP), 148
American College of Allergy and Immunology (ACAI), 148
American Rhinologic Society (ARS), 148-149
Amoxicillin (Amoxil)
  dosage of, 118t, 121, *122-123,* 126-127, 128t, 130t
  indications for, 124t
  susceptibility/resistance to, 104t, 124t, 141
Amoxicillin/clavulanate (Augmentin)
  cefixime with, *123,* 127t, 130t
  dosage of, 118t, 121, *122,* 126, 128t-130t, 132
  against *Haemophilus influenzae,* 101, 103, 104t
  indications for, 124t-126t
  against *Moraxella catarrhalis,* 103
  against *Streptococcus pneumoniae,* 104t, 124t-125t
Anaphylaxis, 79-80
Angiotensin-converting enzyme inhibitors, 31
Animal allergens, extracts for allergy shots, 80
Animal allergies, 28
  control measures for, 40
  seasonal, 25t
  severity of, 28-30
  shots for, 80
  skin tests for, 34
Anosmia, 27, 29
Antibiotics
  frequency of prescriptions for, 11
  resistance to, 97
    alteration of bacterial target or binding site in, 99
    β-lactamase production and, 98-99, 101, *102,* 103
  for rhinosinusitis, 11, 15t, 124t-125t
  selection of, nasal endoscopy in, CP3, 108
Anticholinergic side effects, of oral antihistamines, 48
Anticholinergics, 44t-45t, 70, 71t, 72
Antigen-presenting cell, 21, *22-23*
Antihistamines. See also specific drugs.
  cost of, 69
  intranasal, 41, 44t-45t, 54-55
    intranasal corticosteroids vs, 56-57
    oral antihistamines vs, 55-56
  oral
    action mechanism of, 25
    advantages of, 45, 48
    as anti-inflammatory agents, 26
    asthma and, 50-51
    cardiac effects of, 49-50, 51t
    classification of, 44t, 45, 48
    comparative trials of, 52-54, 68-69

Antihistamines, oral *(continued)*
duration of action, 48-49
effectiveness of, 43, 45, 45t
intranasal antihistamines vs, 55-56
intranasal corticosteroids vs, 68-69
potency of, 49
safety of, 49-51
sedation from, 48, 50, 51t
side effects of, 48-50
skin tests and, 33-34
in pregnancy, 75, 76t-77t
topical, 73, 75t
Antihypertensive agents, 15t, 31
Anti-immunoglobulin E monoclonal antibody
action mechanism of, 74
effectiveness of, 74-75
Anti-inflammatory drugs, in pregnancy, 76t-77t
Antrochoanal polyp, CP6, 109-110
Apnea in sleep, 27
Aspergillus, 25t
Aspirin sensitivity
asthmatic, 19
nasal polyps and, 15t
in nonallergic rhinitis, 92t
Astelin Nasal Spray. See *Azelastine nasal spray.*
Astemizole (Hismanal)
cardiac side effects of, 49-50
effectiveness of, 53
skin tests and, 33-34
Asthma
antihistamines in, 50-51
aspirin sensitivity in, 19
familial, 27
IgE level in, *36*
methacholine responsiveness in, 18
in pregnancy, 75
rhinitis with
evidence for, 83-87, 84t, *85-86*
symptom frequency in, 18
seasonal allergic rhinitis with, 87
Asthma and Allergy Foundation of America (AAFA), 149
Asthma medications, skin tests and, 34
Atarax. See *Hydroxyzine.*
Atopic dermatitis, 29
Atrovent. See *Ipratropium bromide nasal spray.*
Audiometry, 37
Augmentin. See *Amoxicillin/clavulanate.*
Autumn, environmental allergens in, 25t, 30
Avelox (moxifloxacin). See *Moxifloxacin.*
Azalides, 103, 119t, 127t, 131t
Azatadine (Optimine, Trinalin), 46t
Azelastine HCl (Optivar), 75t

17

Azelastine nasal spray (Astelin Nasal Spray)
as anti-inflammatory agent, 26, 54-55
dosage of, 47t, 56
effectiveness of, 54-56
indications for, 54, 56
loratadine with, 55
oral antihistamines vs, 55
in pregnancy, 76t-77t
safety of, 51t
sedation from, 51t
Azithromycin (Zithromax), 119t
in β-lactam allergic patients, 121, 128t-129t, 132
in children, 128t-129t
indications for, 124t
susceptibility/resistance to, 104t, 124t

B cells, *22*
Bacteria, translocation into sinus cavities, 97
Bacterial rhinosinusitis, acute (ABRS). See also *Rhinosinusitis; Sinusitis.*
antibiotic resistance in, 98-99, 101, 103, 104t-105t
computed tomography of, CP7
cost of, 94
diagnosis of, 11-12
maxillary sinus puncture in, 108
maxillary toothache in, 107
nasal endoscopy in, CP2, CP3, 108
nasal secretions in, 10795
plain radiographs in, 108-109
symptoms in, 107
ultrasound in, 108
duration of, 92, 94
epidemiology of, 94
incidence of, 94
orbital invasion by, CP11, 142, *143-144*
pathogens in, 97, *98-99*
recurrent, 94
symptoms of, CP11, 141-142
treatment of, 117, 139-140. See also specific drugs and drug types.
surgical, 142
unilateral, computed tomography of, *105*
from viral rhinitis, 11-12, 96-97, 140
Bactrim. See *Trimethoprim/sulfamethoxazole (TMP/SMX).*
Beclomethasone nasal spray (Beconase AQ, Vancenase)
actions of
duration of, 61
onset of, 61, 65t
classification of, 44t
clinical trials of, 66-67
dosage and delivery of, 62t
effectiveness of, 55, 67-68
pharmacokinetics of, 65t
potency of, 61, 63t
in pregnancy, 76t-77t

Beconase AQ. See *Beclomethasone nasal spray.*
Bed covers, in dust mite avoidance, 40t, 41
Benadryl (diphenhydramine)
  classification of, 45
  dosage of, 46t
  duration of action, 48
  in pregnancy, 76t-77t
Benzalkonium, 74
β-blockers, 31
β-lactam antibiotics, allergic reactions to, 132-133
β-lactamase production, 98-99, 101, *102,* 103
Biaxin. See *Clarithromycin.*
Biologic allergy units (BAU), 35
Birth control pills, 31
Blood pressure medications, 15t, 31
Blood tests
  advantages of, 35-36
  for IgE, 35, *36*
  in rhinitis diagnosis, 35-36
Brompheniramine (Dimetane)
  classification of, 45
  dosage of, 46t
  duration of action, 48
  effectiveness of, 52
  in pregnancy, 76t-77t
  sedation from, 52
Bronchodilators, 76t-77t
Budesonide nasal spray (Rhinocort AQ), 44t
  advantage of, 64
  in children, 64
  comparative trials of, 66-68
  dosage of, 62t, 66-67
  omalizumab with, 88
  onset of action, 65t
  pharmacokinetics of, 65t, 66-67
  potency of, 63t, 64
  in pregnancy, 76t-77t

Cat allergen
  in allergic rhinitis, 144
  extract for allergy shots, 80
Cefdinir (Omnicef)
  for ABRS, 121, *122,* 124t, 128t, 132
  dosage of, 118t
  against *Haemophilus influenzae,* 101, 103, 104t
  against *Moraxella catarrhalis,* 103
  penicillin cross-reactivity with, 132-133
  against *Streptococcus pneumoniae,* 104t
Cefixime (Suprax), 103
  amoxicillin or clindamycin with, *123,* 127t, 130t
Cefpodoxime (Vantin)
  in children, 128t
  dosage of, 118t, 121

17

Cefpodoxime (Vantin) *(continued)*
indications for, 101, 103, *122,* 124t
in penicillin intolerance, 132
susceptibility/resistance to, 101, 103, 104t, 124t
Ceftin (cefuroxime). See *Cefuroxime.*
Ceftriaxone (Rocephin)
for ABRS, *122,* 124t-126t, 128t-129t
in children, 128t-129t
dosage of, 119t
susceptibility/resistance to, 104t
Cefuroxime (Ceftin)
in children, 121, 128t
dosage of, 118t, 121
indications for, *122,* 124t
in penicillin intolerance, 132-133
susceptibility/resistance to, 104t, 124t
Cephalosporins, drug cross-reactivity with, 132-133
Cetirizine (Zyrtec)
for allergic rhinitis, 53
with asthma, 51, 87
as anti-inflammatory agent, 26
classification of, 45
dosage of, 47t
duration of action, 49
effectiveness of, 53-54
potency of, 49
in pregnancy, 76t-77t
safety of, 51t
sedation from, 48, 51t, 53
Children
ABRS in, 12
complications of, 142
drugs for, 117, 120t, 121, 128t-131t, 132
frequency of, 94
pathogens causing, 97, *99*
adenoid hypertrophy in, 13, 27
allergic asthma in, 41
allergic conjunctivitis in, 74
allergic rhinitis in, 16, 37, 72
antihistamine dosages in, oral, 46t-47t
β-lactam allergy in, 128t-129t
corticosteroid nasal sprays in, 64, 66
eczema in, adult atopic dermatitis and, 29
olopatadine in, 74
otitis media in, 37
resources for, 148-149
rhinosinusitis in, diagnosis of, 107, 109
Chlorpheniramine (Chlor-Trimeton)
classification of, 45
dosage of, 46t, 53
duration of action, 48
potency of, 49
in pregnancy, 76t-77t

Ciliary dyskinesia, 28t
Cladosporium, 25t, 31
Clarinex. See *Desloratadine.*
Clarithromycin (Biaxin)
in β-lactam allergy, 128t-129t, 132
dosage of, 119t
effectiveness of, 121
indications for, 124t
susceptibility/resistance to, 105t, 124t
Claritin. See *Loratadine.*
Clavulanate. See *Amoxicillin/clavulanate.*
Clemastine fumarate (Tavist), 47t
Cleocin. See *Clindamycin.*
Clindamycin (Cleocin)
action mechanism of, *106*
cefixime with, *123,* 127t, 130t
in children, 129t
dosage of, 119t
penicillin and, 103t
potency of, 131t
resistance to, 101, 103t
rifampin with, 124t-125t, 127t, 129t-130t
Clinical trials
of beclomethasone, 67
of intranasal antihistamines, 55-57
of intranasal corticosteroids, 56-57, 66-69
of oral antihistamines, 52-56, 68-69
Cockroaches, 25t
Colds, course and resolution of, 13
Computed tomography
in chronic rhinosinusitis, 136t, 137, *138*
in loss of sense of smell/taste, 27
of sinus air-fluid levels, CP8, CP9, 139
of sinus opacification, CP9, 140-141, *143-144*
in sinusitis diagnosis, 109-110, *111-115*
Concha bullosa, 13, 92t
Congenital abnormalities, chronic rhinosinusitis and, 135
Congestion. See *Nasal congestion.*
Conjunctivitis
allergic, 28
vernal
cromolyn ophthalmic drops for, 74
ketotifen for, 75t
Contact lenses, 74
Corticosteroid nasal sprays, 44t-45t
action mechanism of, 25, 60-61
adverse effects of, 64, 66
in children, 64, 66
clinically distinguishing factors of, 65t
comparative trials of, 66-69
cost of, 69
dosage, 62t
duration of action, 44t

Corticosteroid nasal sprays *(continued)*
frequency of prescriptions for, 11
indications for, 43, 69
intranasal antihistamines vs, 56-57
leukotriene receptor antagonists vs, 72-73
potency of, 26, 45t, 63t, 64
selection among, 69
skin tests and, 34
Cost of chronic rhinitis, 11
Cromolyn sodium ophthalmic drops (Opticrom), 74, 75t
Cromolyn sodium solution (Nasalcrom), 44t
for allergic rhinitis, 45t, 70
for chronic rhinitis, 39, 43
for congestion, 26
dosage and delivery of, 44t, 70, 71t
effectiveness of, 45t, 70
in pregnancy, 76t-77t
safety of, 70
Cyproheptadine (Periactin), 47t
Cystic fibrosis, nasal polyps in, 13
Cytokines, agents against, 7871

Decongest. See *Oxymetazoline nasal spray.*
Decongestants
as hybrid, 44t, 59t
as nasal sprays
action mechanism of, 57
classification of, 44t
dosage of, 58t-59t
rebound congestion from, 31, 57
recommended duration of use, 57
oral, 44t
contraindications to, 60
dosage of, 59t
side effects of, 57, 60
withdrawal symptoms from, 60
over-the-counter, dosage and delivery of, 58t-59t
relative effectiveness of, 45t
rhinitis medicamentosa from, 15t, 92t
topical, 15t, 57
Dermatitis, atopic, 29
childhood eczema and, 29
IgE level in, *36*
Desloratadine (Clarinex)
for asthma, 87
classification of, 45t, 48
clinical trials of, 54-55
distinguishing properties of, 54
dosage of, 47t
duration of action, 49
indications for, 52
pharmacokinetics of, 51
potency of, 49

Desloratadine (Clarinex) *(continued)*
in pregnancy, 76t-77t
safety of, 51t, 51-52
Dexamethasone nasal spray, 44t, 61, 64, 65t
Diagnosis and Management of Rhinitis: Parameter Documents of the Joint Task Force on Practice Parameters in Allergy, Asthma, and Immunology, 37
Dimetane. See *Brompheniramine.*
Diphenhydramine (Benadryl)
classification of, 45
dosage of, 46t
duration of action, 48
in pregnancy, 76t-77t
Doxycycline (Vibramycin)
in ABRS, 124t, 127t
action mechanism of, 106t
in β-lactam allergy, 121, *123,* 127t
dosage of, 120t
penicillin and, 103t
resistance to, 101, 103t, 105t
Dristan Long-Lasting. See *Oxymetazoline nasal spray.*
Dristan Nasal (phenylephrine HCl/pheniramine maleate), 59t
Duration. See *Phenylephrine nasal spray.*
Dust mite allergen
control measures for, 40t, 40-41, 145
extract for allergy shots, 80
seasonal, 25t
skin tests for, 34
vacuuming and, 30-31

Eardrum ventilating tubes, 37
Eczema, childhood, adult atopic dermatitis and, 29
Efedron Gel (ephedrine), 58t, 60
Endocrine rhinitis, 92t
Endoscopic sinus surgery, computer-aided, 137, *138*
Endoscopy, nasal. See *Nasal endoscopy.*
Environmental allergens, seasonal, 25t, 28t, 30-31, 92t, 142-145. See also *Allergens.*
Environmental chemicals/pollutants, chronic rhinosinusitis and, 135
Environmental control
in allergy avoidance, 40t, 40-41
in chronic rhinitis, 15t
Enzyme-linked immunosorbent assay (ELISA), for IgE, 35-36
Eosinophil(s), in inflammatory cascade, 21-22, *22-23*
Eosinophil count, 33
Eosinophilia
in nonallergic rhinitis. See *Nonallergic rhinitis with eosinophilia syndrome.*
in rhinitis syndromes, 14t
Ephedrine (Efedron gel), 58t, 60
Epinephrine nasal spray, 44t
Epistaxis, 63-64, 67-68

Erythromycin
for ABRS, 128t-129t
in β-lactam allergy, 132
indications for, 121, 124t
stomach intolerance to, 140
susceptibility/resistance to, 105t, 124t
Ethanolamines, 46t
Ethmoid sinuses
anatomy of, CP1, 95, *96*
diseased, CP7, 139
opacification of, CP7, *143-144*
surgical drainage of, 142
Exercise, for vasomotor instability, 15t
Expectorants, iodide-containing, 75
Eyes
itchy, 28, 45
treatment of, 73-74, 75t

Facial pain, 139
Factive (gemifloxacin), 105t, 120t
Fall, environmental allergens in, 25t, 30
Familial disorders, 29
Family history, 15t
Fexofenadine (Allegra)
azelastine with, 55-56
classification of, 45, 48
dosage of, 47t
duration of action, 49
effectiveness of, 50, 52-53, 55-56
potency of, 49
in pregnancy, 76t-77t
safety of, 50, 51t
sedation from, 48, 51t
Flonase. See *Fluticasone nasal spray.*
Flunisolide nasal spray (Nasalide, Nasarel), 44t
action of
duration of, 61
onset of, 65t
dosage of, 62t
pharmacokinetics of, 65t
potency of, 63t
in pregnancy, 76t-77t
Fluoroquinolones, against *Streptococcus pneumoniae* and *Haemophilus influenzae,* 101, 103, 105t, *106,* 123t, 126t
Fluticasone nasal spray (Flonase), 44t
adverse effects of, 63
in children, 64
comparative trials of, 66-68, 72
dosage of, 62t
indications for, 61
onset of action, 61, 65t
pharmacokinetics of, 65t
potency of, 61, 63t, 63-64
in pregnancy, 76t-77t

Folate inhibitors, 104t, 119t. See also *Trimethoprim/ sulfamethoxazole (TMP/SMX).*
Food allergy
rhinitis from, 31
skin tests for, 34
Foradil, 76t-77t
Foreign body, 28t
4-Way Fast-Acting, 59t
Frontal sinuses, anatomy of, CP1, 95
Fungus, chronic rhinosinusitis and, 135
Fusarium, 25t

Gatifloxacin (Tequin)
dosage of, 120t
indications for, 121, *122,* 125t
susceptibility/resistance to, 105t, 124t-127t
Gemifloxacin (Factive), 105t, 120t
Genetic abnormalities, chronic rhinosinusitis and, 135
Geographic locations, allergen variation in, 30
Granulocyte-macrophage colony-stimulating factor, in early- and late-phase allergic response, 26
Granulomatous disease, in nasal obstruction, 27, 28t, 92t
Grass pollen allergen
extract for allergy shots, 80
seasonal, 25t, 30, 143-144
Guanethidine, rhinitis from, 31
Gustatory rhinitis, 18

Haemophilus influenzae
antibiotic resistance/susceptibility of, 99, 101, 103, 104t, 124t-125t, 127t, 129t
β-lactamase production by, 99, *102,* 103
as rhinosinusitis pathogen, 97, *98-99*
Headache, 29
Heart, antihistamine adverse effects on, 49-50, 51t
High-efficiency particulate air (HEPA) filters, 41
Hismanal. See *Astemizole.*
Histamine, symptoms triggered by, 26
Horner's syndrome, 92t
Hybrid intranasal spray, 44t, 59t
Hydrocortisone potency, 63t
Hydroxyzine (Atarax, Vistaril)
classification of, 45, 48
dosage of, 46t
duration of action, 48
sedation from, 48
skin tests and, 33-34
Hypothyroidism, rhinitis and, 92t

Idiopathic rhinitis, 92t
Immunodeficiency, chronic rhinosinusitis in, 135

17

Immunoglobulin E (IgE). See also *Anti-immunoglobulin E monoclonal antibody; Omalizumab.*
allergic rhinitis and, 16
aspirin sensitivity and, 19
in asthma, *86*
blood tests for, 35, *36*
in chronic rhinitis syndromes, 14t
to environmental allergen, 33
in inflammatory cascade, 21-22, *22-24*
overlap in allergic diseases, *36*
Immunotherapy
action mechanism of, 79-80
advantages of, 25
allergy skin test extracts for, 35
anaphylaxis in, 79-80
for chronic rhinitis, 15t
for congestion, 26
dosages in, 80-81
effectiveness of, 79
goals of, 81
indications for, 79
interval between shots in, 81
omalizumab added to, 88
In vitro assays. See *Blood tests.*
Infectious rhinitis, 92t
Inflammatory cascade, in allergic rhinitis, 21-22, *22-24,* 24-26
Interleukins
agents against, 78
in early- and late-phase allergic response, *24,* 26
in inflammatory cascade, 21-22, *23*
Iodides, in expectorants, 75
Ipratropium bromide nasal spray (Atrovent), 44t
action mechanism of, 70
dosage of, 71t, 72
effectiveness of, 70
onset of action, 70
for rhinitis, 44t
Itching
nasal. See *Nasal itching.*
ocular, 28, 45

Keratoconjunctivitis, 74
Ketek (telithromycin)
for ABRS, 121, *123,* 124t
dosage of, 119t
resistance/susceptibility to, 103, 104t
Ketolides
for ABRS, 119t, 127t
action mechanism of, 106t
resistance to, 101
susceptibility/resistance to, 101, 104t
Ketorolac tromethamine (Acular), 74, 75t
Ketotifen fumarate (Zaditor), 74, 75t, 78
Kinins, symptoms triggered by, 25

Laboratory tests, in rhinitis diagnosis, 33-36
Leukotriene receptor antagonists
  future of, 78
  in treating allergic rhinitis, 44t-45t, 72-73, 145
Leukotrienes
  azelastine and, 55
  in early and late phase allergic response, *24*
  symptoms triggered by, 25
Levaquin. See *Levofloxacin.*
Levocabastine (Livostin), 56, 73-74, 75t
Levofloxacin (Levaquin)
  for ABRS, 124t-127t
  in β-lactam allergy, 125t
  dosage of, 120t
  indications for, 121, *122,* 125t
  susceptibility/resistance to, 105t, 125t
Livostin (levocabastine), 56, 73-74, 75t
Lodoxamide, 74
Loratadine (Claritin)
  for allergic rhinitis, 51, 87
  as anti-inflammatory agent, 26
  for asthma, 51, 87
  azelastine with, 55
  classification of, 45, 48
  clinical trials of, 52-55
  dosage of, 47t
  duration of action, 49
  effectiveness of, 51-54
  potency of, 49
  in pregnancy, 76t-77t
  safety of, 50, 51t
  sedation from, 48, 51t
Loteprednol (Alrex), 75t

Macrolides
  dosages of, 119t
  in penicillin intolerance, 127t
  resistance to, 101, 103, 104t-105t
Macrophage, in inflammatory cascade, 21, *22-23*
Magnetic resonance imaging, in chronic rhinosinusitis, 136t, 137
Major basic protein, *23*
Malignant tumors, nasal, 27
Mast cell
  degranulation of, 24
  in early- and late-phase allergic response, *24*
  in inflammatory cascade, 21-22, *22-23,* 24
Maxillary sinuses
  air-fluid level in, CP4, 108
  anatomy of, CP1, 95, *96*
  opacification of, CP5, CP9, 141, *143*
Medical history, 27-28
Medication history, 31
Metaproterenol, 76t-77t

17

Methacholine challenge, 18, 86, 88, 145
Methyldopa, 31
Mold allergy
  indoors, 25t
  outdoors, 25t, 31, 40
  seasonal, 25t, 31
  skin tests for, 34
  spore count in, 25t, 31
Mometasone nasal spray (Nasonex), 44t, 61
  in children, 64
  comparative trials of, 66-68
  dosage of, 62t
  duration of action, 61
  onset of action, 61, 65t
  pharmacokinetics of, 65t
  potency of, 61, 64, 65t
  in pregnancy, 76t-77t
Monoclonal antibody, against IgE, 74-75. See also *Omalizumab.*
Montelukast (Singulair), 44t
  action mechanism of, 72
  in children, 72
  dosage of, 71t
  effectiveness of, 72-74, 87
  intranasal steroid sprays vs, 72-73
  pharmacokinetics of, 72
  in pregnancy, 76t-77t
  safety of, 73
Moraxella catarrhalis
  antibiotic resistance/susceptibility of, 99, 101, 103
  β-lactamase production by, 99, 101, 103
  as rhinosinusitis pathogen, 97, *98-99*
Moxifloxacin (Avelox)
  dosage of, 120t, 121, *122*
  effectiveness of, 126t
  indications for, 124t-125t
  susceptibility/resistance to, 105t, *123,* 125t
Mucociliary dysfunction, chronic rhinosinusitis and, 135
Mucosa
  edema of, 57
  inflammation of, in polyposis etiology, 19
  in NARES, 33
Mucosal barrier, inhaled allergen penetration of, 21
MYCl Spray, 59t

Naphazoline for eyes, 73
Naphazoline nasal spray (Privine)
  dosage of, 58t-59t
  duration of action, 44t, 58t
  in hybrid intranasal spray, 59t
  rebound congestion from, 57
NARES. See *Nonallergic rhinitis with eosinophilia syndrome.*
Nasacort. See *Triamcinolone acetonide nasal spray.*
Nasal bleeding, 63-64, 67-68

Nasal congestion
drugs for, 26. See also *Decongestants.*
pathophysiology of, 57
polyps and, 28-29
rebound, 31, 57
in rhinitis syndromes, 14t
in sleep disturbance, 27
triggers of, 25
Nasal discharge
drugs for, 45t
in upper respiratory infections, 92
in various disorders, 33
Nasal drainage, in chronic rhinosinusitis, CP10, 141
Nasal endoscopy, CP3, 27
in ABRS diagnosis, 108
in anatomic obstruction diagnosis, 32
in chronic rhinosinusitis diagnosis, 135, 136t
with Gram's stain, in detecting sinus bacteria, 97
Nasal itching
in allergic rhinitis, 28
oral antihistamines for, 45, 48
triggers of, 26
Nasal obstruction
causes of, 27
fluctuations in, 27
in rhinitis. See *Structural rhinitis.*
Nasal patency, 31
Nasal polyps
age and, 13, 15t, 19
allergy skin tests and, 19
antrochoanal, CP6, 109-110
asthmatic aspirin sensitivity in, 19
computed tomography of, *114*
corticosteroid nasal sprays for, 69
detection of, 32
etiology of, 19
factors associated with, 15t
incidence of, 19, 27
nasal congestion and, 28-29
sinus abnormalities and, 19
symptoms of, 14t
systemic corticosteroids for, 19
treatment of, 15t
Nasal saline, 139
for vasomotor instability, 15t
Nasal septal deformity. See *Septal deviation.*
Nasal septum, anatomy of, *96*
Nasal speculum, 32
Nasal spray. See *Decongestants, as nasal sprays.*
Nasal trauma, structural rhinitis and, 15t
Nasalcrom. See *Cromolyn sodium solution.*
Nasalide. See *Flunisolide nasal spray.*
Nasarel. See *Flunisolide nasal spray.*

Nasonex. See *Mometasone nasal spray.*
National Ambulatory Medical Care Survey, 11
Nedocromil sodium (Alocril), 75t-77t
Neoplasms
  chronic rhinosinusitis and, 135
  detection of, 32
  malignant, 27
  rhinitis from, 92t
Neo-Synephrine. See *Oxymetazoline nasal spray; Phenylephrine nasal spray.*
Nitric oxide, in paranasal sinuses, 96
Nonallergic rhinitis, 92t
Nonallergic rhinitis with eosinophilia syndrome (NARES), 92t
  age at onset, 15t
  factors associated with, 15t
  nasal discharge in, 33
  symptoms of, 14t, 16, 18
  treatment of, 15t
Norastemizole, 50, 54, 78
Northern United States, seasonal allergens in, 25t
Nose
  endoscopy of. See *Nasal endoscopy.*
  physical examination of, 32-33
Nostril. See *Phenylephrine.*
Nostrilla. See *Oxymetazoline nasal spray.*
Novafed (pseudoephedrine), 44t, 59t
  dosage and delivery of, 59t
  side effects of, 57, 60

Occupational irritants. See *Workplace.*
Ocular itching, 28, 45
Ocular therapy, 73-74, 75t
Olive allergen, 30
Olopatadine (Patanol), 74, 75t, 78
Omalizumab (Xolair)
  added to immunotherapy, 88
  for allergic rhinitis, 87-89
  for asthma, 74, 88
  dosage of, 87, 89
  subcutaneous, 88-89
Omnicef. See *Cefdinir.*
Opacification, of sinuses, CP5, CP7, CP9, 140-141, *143-144*
Opticrom (cromolyn sodium ophthalmic drops), 74, 75t
Optimine (azatadine), 46t
Optivar (azelastine HCl), 75t
Oral contraceptives, rhinitis medicamentosa from, 31
Orbital abscess, from ABRS, CP11, 142, *143-144*
Ostiomeatal complex, normal, *96*
Ostiomeatal obstruction, CP7
Otitis media, 37
Otrivin (xylometazoline nasal spray)
  congestion from, 57
  dosage of, 58t
  duration of action, 44t, 58t

Oxymetazoline nasal spray (Afrin, Decongest, Dristan Long-Lasting, Neo-Synephrine, Nostrilla), 57
dosage of, 58t
duration of action, 44t, 58t
rebound congestion from, 57, 61

Patanol (olopatadine), 74, 75t
Patency, nasal, 31
Pemirolast potassium (Alamast), 75t
Penicillin
for ABRS, 142
action mechanism of, 106t
cross-reactivity with cephalosporins, 132-133
cross-resistance with other antibiotic classes, 103t
intolerance to, 132
Streptococcus pneumoniae resistance to, 99, 101, *102,* 104t-105t, *123*
Penicillin binding proteins, 101
Penicillium, 25t
Periactin (cyproheptadine), 47t
Phenergan (promethazine), 46t
Pheniramine maleate, 59t, 73
Phentolamine, 31
Phenylephrine HCl/naphazoline HCl/pyrilamine maleate (4-Way Fast-Acting), 59t
Phenylephrine HCl/pheniramine maleate (Dristan Nasal), 59t
Phenylephrine HCl/pyrilamine maleate (MYCl Spray), 59t
Phenylephrine nasal spray (Duration, Neo-Synephrine, Nostril, Vicks-Sinex)
classification of, 44t
dosage of, 58t
duration of action, 58t
in hybrid sprays, 59t
rebound congestion from, 31, 57
Phenylpropanolamine, 60
Physical examination, 32-33
Piperazines, 46t
Pollen allergens
extracts of for allergy shots, 80
outdoors, 40
seasonal, 28t, 30, 92t
by geographic location, 30
from trees, 25t, 30, 80
skin tests for, 34
in differential diagnosis, 92t
Polyps, nasal. See *Nasal polyps.*
Postnasal drainage, 14t
Prazosin, 31
Prednisone, 76t-77t
Pregnancy
asthma/allergy medications in, 75, 76t-77t
rhinitis in, 28t, 31, 92t
vasomotor instability and, 15t

Privine (naphazoline nasal spray)
  dosage of, 58t-59t
  duration of action, 44t, 58t
  rebound congestion from, 57
Promethazine (Phenergan), 46t
Prostaglandins, 25
Protein nitrogen units (PNU), 35
Pruritus, 29
Pseudoephedrine (Novafed, Pseudogest, Sudafed), 44t
  dosage and delivery of, 59t
  side effects of, 57, 60
Pseudogest (pseudoephedrine), 44t
  dosage and delivery of, 59t
  side effects of, 57, 60
Pyrilamine maleate, in hybrid intranasal spray, 59t

QT interval, antihistamines and, 49-50
Quinolones, 120t

Radioallergosorbent test (RAST), 35-36
Radiography
  in chronic rhinosinusitis, 137t
  in sinus air-fluid level determination, CP4, 108-109
  in sinusitis diagnosis, 108-109, *110*
Ragweed allergen, 16, 25t
  beclomethasone trial in, 67
  comparative antihistamine effectiveness against, 53-54, 67
  extract of, for allergy shots, 80
  in skin tests, 35
Reserpine, rhinitis from, 31
Resources for allergy/asthma, 147-149
Respiratory infection, viral. See *Viral upper respiratory infection.*
Rhinitis. See also *Rhinosinusitis.*
  allergic. See *Allergic rhinitis.*
  asthma coexistence with, 27
    evidence for, 83-87, 84t, *85-86*
  chronic
    anatomy and, 13
    asthma in, 27
    disorders in, 13, 14t-15t
  complications of, 36-37
  definition of, 11, 13
  diagnosis of
    blood tests in, 35-36
    medical history in, 27-28
    medication history in, 31
    mold spore counts in, 31
    physical examination in, 32-33
    seasonal pollen counts in, 30-31
    skin tests in, 14t, 33-35
    symptoms and signs in, 28t, 29-30
  differential diagnosis of, 28t
  endocrine, 92t

Rhinitis *(continued)*
idiopathic, 92t
IgE level in, *36*
medication-induced, 31
pathogenesis of, 21-26
in pregnancy, 31
secondary, 28t, 92t
treatment of. See *Rhinitis treatment.*
types of, 14t-15t, 92t. See also specific type, eg, *Allergic rhinitis; Structural rhinitis.*
in differential diagnosis, 28t
Rhinitis medicamentosa, 28t, 92t
age at onset, 15t
from decongestant nasal spray, 57
factors associated with, 15t
symptoms of, 14t
treatment of, 15t
Rhinitis treatment, 15t
avoidance of allergens as, 39-40, 40t
goals of, 12, 39
immunotherapy in, 79-81
pharmacologic. See also specific drugs or drug types.
anticholinergics in, 44t-45t, 70, 71t, 72
corticosteroids in, 43, 44t-45t, 60-61, 63, 65t, 66-69
cromolyn sodium in, 43, 44t-45t, 70, 71t
decongestants in, 43, 44t-45t, 57, 60
in future, 78
inhaled antihistamines in, 43, 44t-45t, 54-55
ocular, 73-74, 75t
oral antihistamines in, 43, 44t-47t, 45, 48-54, 54-55
in pregnancy, 75
Rhinocort AQ. See *Budesonide nasal spray.*
Rhinorrhea
in rhinitis syndromes, 14t, 29
triggers of, 25-26
Rhinoscopy, in loss of sense of smell/taste, 27
Rhinosinusitis. See also *Rhinitis; Sinusitis.*
acute bacterial. See *Bacterial rhinosinusitis, acute.*
age at onset, 15t
chronic
computed tomography of, CP7
diagnosis of, 135136t-137t
duration of, 136t
imaging in, 136t-137t, 137
nasal drainage in, CP10, 141
surgery for, 137, *138*
treatment of, 141
classification of, 91-92, 93t
definition of, 11, 91
differential diagnosis of, 92t
factors associated with, 15t
incidence of, 11
nasal discharge in, 33, 108

17

Rhinosinusitis *(continued)*
symptoms of, 14t
treatment of, 15t, 110, 117. See also specific drugs and drug types.
antibiotics in, 11, 15t, 111, 117, 124t-125t
goals of, 12
triggers of, 91
viral, 11, 91-92, 92t
Rifampin
clindamycin with, 124t-125t, 127t, 129t-130t
drug interactions with, 127t
TMP/SMX with, 129t
Rocephin. See *Ceftriaxone.*

Saline, nasal, 139
Salmeterol, 76t-77t
Seasonal variations
in environmental allergens, 25t, 28t, 30-31, 92t
in pollen count, 28t, 30, 92t
in rhinitis syndromes, 14t
Sedation, 48, 50, 51t
Seldane (terfenadine)
cardiac side effects of, 49-50
effectiveness of, 52-54
for ocular itching, 74
Sense of smell/taste, loss of, 27, 29
Septal deviation, 13
computed tomography of, *112*
detection of, 32
incidence of, 27
in structural rhinitis, 27, 28t, 92t
Septal perforation, 64
Septal spur, *113*
Septra. See *Trimethoprim/sulfamethoxazole (TMP/SMX).*
Septum, anatomy of, *96*
Sinex (xylometazoline nasal spray)
dosage of, 58t
duration of action, 44t, 58t
rebound congestion from, 57
Singulair. See *Montelukast.*
Sinus(es)
air-fluid levels in, CP4, CP7, CP8, CP9, 139, 141
anatomy of, CP1, 95, *96*
computed tomography of
of bilateral sinusitis, *115*
of deviated septum, *112*
normal, *111*
of polyp, *114*
of septal spur, *113*
development of, 95
functions of, 95-96
maxillary
air fluid level in, *110*
polyp in, *114*
opacification of, CP5, CP7, CP9, 140-141

Sinus and Allergy Health Partnership (SAHP), 149
Sinusitis, 92t. See also *Bacterial rhinosinusitis, acute; Rhinosinusitis.*
asthma and chronic rhinitis from, 85
bilateral, computed tomography of, *106*
chronic, asthma in, 27
diagnosis of, computed tomography in, 109-110, *115*
Sinusoids, venous, engorgement of, 57
Skin tests. See *Allergy skin tests.*
Sleep apnea, 27
Smell, losing sense of, 27-29
Smoke exposure
asthma symptoms and, 41
chronic rhinosinusitis and, 135
Sneezing
in rhinitis syndromes, 14t, 29
treatment of, 45t
triggers of, 25
Soft tissue, in nasal obstruction, 27
Sphenoid sinuses, CP1, 95
Spring, environmental allergens in, 25t, 30
Staphylococcus aureus
as ABRS pathogen, 97, *98*
β-lactamase production by, 99
Staphylococcus pyogenes, as ABRS pathogen, 97, *99*
Steroids. See *Corticosteroid nasal spray.*
Streptococcus pneumoniae
as ABRS pathogen, 97, *98-99*
antibiotic susceptibility of, 97, 99, 101, 103, 104t-105t, 124t-125t, 127t, 129t
penicillin-resistant, *102*
other antibiotic class cross-resistance in, 103t
Streptococcus pyogenes, 97
Structural rhinitis
adenoidal hypertrophy in, 27
age at onset, 15t
factors associated with, 15t
nasal polyps in, 27. See also *Nasal polyps.*
septal deformity in. See *Septal deviation.*
symptoms of, 14t
treatment of, 15t
Sudafed (pseudoephedrine), 44t
dosage and delivery of, 59t
side effects of, 57, 60
Summer, environmental allergens in, 25t, 30
Sympathomimetics. See *Corticosteroid nasal spray.*

Taste, losing sense of, 27, 29
Tavist (clemastine fumarate), 47t
Telithromycin (Ketek)
for ABRS, 121, *123,* 124t
dosage of, 119t
resistance/susceptibility to, 103, 104t

Tequin (gatifloxacin)
  dosage of, 120t
  indications for, 105t, 124t-127t
  susceptibility/resistance to, 105t
Terbutaline, 76t-77t
Terfenadine (Seldane)
  cardiac side effects of, 49-50
  effectiveness of, 52-54
  for ocular itching, 74
Tetracycline, 75, 105t, *106,* 120t
Tetrahydrozoline nasal spray (Tyzine)
  dosage of, 58t
  duration of action, 44t, 58t
T-helper cell
  in early- and late-phase allergic response, 26
  in inflammatory cascade, 21-22, *22-24*
Theophylline, 76t-77t
Thyroid disorders
  rhinitis in, 92t
  vasomotor instability and, 15t
TMP/SMX. See *Trimethoprim/sulfamethoxazole.*
Toothache, maxillary, 107
Torsade de pointes, 49
Tree pollen allergens
  for allergy shots, 80
  seasonal, 25t, 28-30
Triamcinolone acetonide nasal spray (Nasacort, Tri-Nasal Spray), 44t
  action of
    duration of, 61, 63
    onset of, 65t
  comparative trials of, 66-68
  dosage of, 62t
  pharmacokinetics of, 65t
  potency of, 63t
  in pregnancy, 76t-77t
Trimethoprim/sulfamethoxazole (TMP/SMX) (Bactrim, Septra)
  action mechanism of, 106t
  in β-lactam allergy, 131t, 132
  in children, 128t
  dosage of, 119t
  penicillin and, 103t
  in penicillin intolerance, 127t
  resistance to, 101, 103
  rifampin with, 129t
Trinalin (azatadine), 46t
Tri-Nasal Spray (triamcinolone acetonide). See *Triamcinolone acetonide nasal spray.*
Triprolidine, 76t-77t
Tumor necrosis factor-α
  in early- and late-phase allergic response, *24,* 25
  symptoms triggered by, 25

Turbinates
abnormalities of, 92t
anatomy of, CP1, 95, *96*
appearance of, 32
size of, 13
Tylenol Allergy Sinus, 144
Tympanic membrane, in otitis media, 37
Tyzine (tetrahydrozoline nasal spray)
dosage of, 58t
duration of action, 44t, 58t

Ultrasonography, in rhinosinusitis diagnosis, 108
Upper respiratory infection
duration of
bacterial, 92, 94
viral, 91-92, 92t, 117
rhinosinusitis and, 15t
viral
duration of, 91, 117
rhinosinusitis and, 11
Urinary retention, 48, 60

Vancenase. See *Beclomethasone nasal spray.*
Vantin (cefpodoxime)
dosage of, 118t
indications for, 124t
susceptibility/resistance to, 104t, 124t
Vasoactive chemicals, 31
Vasomotor instability, 14t-15t
Vasomotor rhinitis, 16, 92t
Vibramycin. See *Doxycycline.*
Vicks-Sinex. See *Phenylephrine nasal spray.*
Viral rhinitis, 92t
computed tomography in, 109
course and resolution of, 13
decongestants for, 57
duration of, 92, 94
nasal discharge in, 32-33, 92
Viral upper respiratory infection
ABRS from, 11-12, 96-97, 139-140
duration of, 91, 117
rhinosinusitis after, 11, 91, 92t, 96
Vistaril. See *Hydroxyzine.*

Wegener granulomatosis, in nasal obstruction, 27, 28t, 92t
Winter, environmental allergens in, 25t, 30
Workplace
inhalant allergies in, 17t
irritants in, 17t
lost time at, from chronic rhinitis/sinusitis, 11

Xolair. See *Omalizumab.*
Xylometazoline nasal spray (Otrivin, Sinex)
  dosage of, 58t
  duration of action, 44t, 58t
  rebound congestion from, 57

Zaditor (ketotifen fumarate), 74, 75t, 78
Zafirlukast, 76t-77t
Zileuton, 76t-77t, 78
Zithromax (azithromycin), 119t
  in β-lactam allergy, 121, 128t-129t, 132
  in children, 128t-129t
  indications for, 121, 124t
  susceptibility/resistance to, 104t, 124t
Zyrtec. See *Cetirizine.*